Praise for Run Your Butt Off!

"I used to hate to run. I hated it just like most of the kids in gym class. Running the mile felt like an eternity. If you would have told me then that one day I would run in the Olympic marathon and be running 15 to 20 miles a day in training and loving every minute of it, I would have laughed. The most difficult step that all of us take in running is the first step, whether it's the first step of beginning training or the first step of a marathon race. One of the keys to getting through that first step of training is to break running down into manageable bite-size pieces, which is exactly what *Run Your Butt Off!* has done. This method of training will lead to bigger and bigger breakthroughs in your fitness until one day you might find yourself at the finish of a marathon."

—Ryan Hall, Olympian and American record holder in the half-marathon

"If you want to be more healthy and fit, *Run Your Butt Off!* is the book for you. It will teach you how to make smarter food choices, and it provides an easy-to-follow program that can turn anyone into a runner. *Run Your Butt Off!* is the guide for anyone who wants a healthier lifestyle."

—Rebecca Lobo, Olympic gold medalist and former WNBA player

"I have traveled all over the world. I need to exercise to stay fit for my business. Running has been something I have done from Sweden to Thailand. It's a great way to get out and explore this wonderful world we live in. When you can move and breathe in fresh air while looking at your surroundings during running, you feel strong, powerful, and that all is well. Problems are solved or diminish.

"This book is for people who want to start exercising and do the right thing but don't know how to safely and correctly begin. I started to run at 21, and eight marathons and 30 years later, I can tell you RUNNING IS A GOOD THING! It helps you feel good about yourself both inside and out. So, read this book and then just put one foot in front of the other. And experience our runners' high."

—Kim Alexis, supermodel

Run Your Butt Off!

Run Your Butt Off!

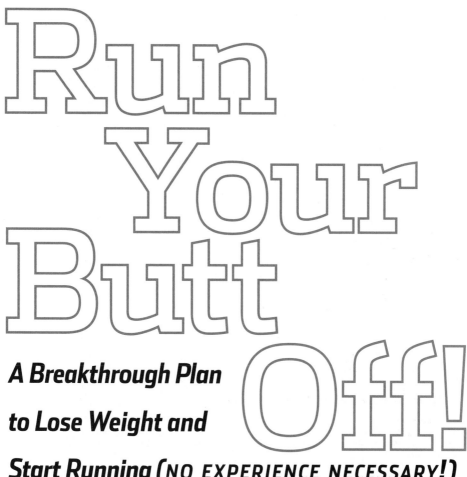

A Breakthrough Plan to Lose Weight and Start Running (NO EXPERIENCE NECESSARY!)

Sarah Lorge Butler with Leslie Bonci, MPH, RD, and

Budd Coates, MS, the *Runner's World* running coach

RODALE

Direct and trade editions both published in 2011.

© 2011 by Sarah Lorge Butler and Leslie Bonci

Photographs © 2011 by Rodale Inc.

Rodale books may be purchased for business or promotional use or for special sales. For information, please write to:
Special Markets Department, Rodale Inc., 733 Third Avenue, New York, NY 10017

Runner's World is a registered trademark of Rodale Inc.

Printed in the United States of America
Rodale Inc. makes every effort to use acid-free ♾, recycled paper ♺.

Photographs by Tom McDonald
Book design by Christina Gaugler

Library of Congress Cataloging-in-Publication Data

Lorge Butler, Sarah.
   Run your butt off! : a breakthrough plan to lose weight and start running (no experience necessary!) / Sarah Lorge Butler with Leslie Bonci and Budd Coates, Runner's World running coach.
      p.   cm.
   Includes index.
   ISBN-13 978–1–60529–404–9 trade paperback
   ISBN-13 978–1–60961–784–4 direct hardcover
   1. Reducing exercises. 2. Running. I. Bonci, Leslie. II. Coates, Budd. III. Title.
RA781.6.L67 2011
613.7'1—dc22
                                         2010045805

Distributed to the trade by Macmillan
   4 6 8 10 9 7 5 3   trade paperback
2 4 6 8 10 9 7 5 3 1   direct hardcover

www.rodalebooks.com

Contents

Foreword

At the 2010 Chicago Marathon expo, a pair of husband-and-wife runners stop by to introduce themselves. We're chatting, and they appear to be any two middle-aged runners, excited for the race the next day. But as their story unfolds, it slowly dawns on me that I'm seeing a shadow of their former selves. The wife got started running first, and she tells me she has lost 150 pounds.

Say what? One hundred fifty pounds? Can that be? I'm looking at her, trying to imagine what she must have looked like almost double the size. Then the husband chimes in. Motivated by his wife's success, he started running, and now his weight is down 100 pounds. That's more than 250 pounds, *poof,* gone, from one couple. They're proud of themselves, thankful for their newfound health, thrilled with how far they've come, and a little giddy at the possibilities out there for them.

As they should be. I hear stories like that more and more these days. With *Runner's World,* I travel to a lot of races. And these days if there are 50 people at a gathering, it seems at least six will have an incredible weight-loss story. These are folks who tell us they weighed north of 300 pounds a few years ago, before they decided to make a change. They cut back on their calories and started walking on the treadmill. Then the story lines start to sound pretty similar: After a couple of weeks of consistent walking, they break into a jog. Then they push a little longer, running 1 mile, 2 miles, 3. Sometimes they get to the half-marathon—or, in the case of the Chicago couple, the marathon. No matter the distance, they discover more of a life for themselves than they ever thought they'd have.

I'm a competitive runner, and I'll always love the excellence of the elites who run marathons in a little over 2 hours, sustaining what seems like impossible speeds over grueling distances. But maybe I've softened a little in the decades since I won the 1968 Boston Marathon. These days, the stories of people changing their lives through running, losing a lot of weight, and improving their health and fitness touch me so much more. Here are people who, with running, have a whole new outlook. They feel like running has given them a second chance. They'll live to see their grandchildren prosper. These stories get me right in the heart.

All weight-loss experts agree that calorie cutting is the first order of business when you need to shed pounds. Eat less and you'll lose weight. But the long-term route to losing weight is trimming the diet and adding consistent aerobic exercise to keep the pounds off. And for that, running is the best. It's simply the most efficient way to burn calories in the least amount of time.

Any convert to running will tell you that the first steps are the hardest. It takes strength and courage, especially when you're bigger than you want to be, to decide to try running. You've done yourself a favor by picking up this book. The plan in these pages is simple and straightforward. It breaks down running, which might seem impossible right now, into easy, manageable steps, 1 minute at a time.

Give it a try and see where you end up. Enjoy the journey. I won't be shocked if I meet you in a year or two at a race, much thinner, healthier, and happier than your former self. When you get there, be sure to stop by and introduce yourself.

Happy running.

Amby Burfoot
1968 Boston Marathon Champion
Runner's World *Editor at Large*

Introduction

ANYONE CAN BE A RUNNER

You've picked up this book because you want to shed some pounds. Maybe it's 2. Maybe it's 20. Maybe it's way, way more than that.

And you're thinking there's something really freakin' annoying about a bunch of skinny people, the folks who work at *Runner's World,* telling you how great running feels and how if you run, you never have to worry about your weight. "You people don't understand," you're muttering to yourself right now. "You with the fancy watches and the tanned arms and the little running shorts and the cut calves and the furnaces for metabolisms—I don't need any of your sanctimony."

Well, let's get a couple things straight. You're right about the first part. We do love running, and we could talk all day about why. In fact, we often do just that at expos—those trade shows where runners pick up their numbers before big races.

But the second part is where you're mistaken. Not all runners are skinny.

This is not just a sport for the size 2s or the 130-pound guys. Runners, too, exhibit variation in the species. In fact, some races have categories for larger runners, known as Athenas (women who weigh more than 150 pounds) and Clydesdales (men heavier than 200 pounds). Although most elites are tiny, there are exceptions: 1,500-meter Olympian Erin Donohue weighs in at 143 pounds, and she looks strong enough to kick over a truck. Chris Solinsky, who set the American record of 26:59 in the 10,000 meters in 2010, is a big guy by competitive running standards: 6 feet 1 inch and 165 pounds.

Not that they're fat, mind you. Their body fat is next to nothing. But they're bigger than their peers, and they're very successful. So there's room for you to expand your mental image of what a "runner" looks like.

Plus, when it comes to us recreational runners, it is not easy to maintain the weight we want. Almost all of us fret about our size at some time or another. Let me be the first to admit this: I stepped on the scale on Monday, January 4, 2010, and saw a number that was 10 pounds higher than it should have been. I was shocked, but staring back at me in the digital display was a very good explanation for the achiness in my knees, feet, and shins. I was exercising too little, eating too many of the holiday treats I was supposed to be baking for my kids' teachers, and I needed to work at keeping fit. Lifelong runners are not exempt from the upward creep of the scale.

But we also know that given the choice between moving a lot more or eating a lot less, it's more fun to do the former. When running is going well, it does feel great. The miles fly by and the calories are torched, roughly 100 for every mile you run.

Dieting? Well, it's a drag. It's all about deprivation and what you can't have. Cut this, eliminate that. It's about subtraction, saying no.

With running, you're adding a new sport, new friends, and new experiences to your life. You're engaging in something human beings have

> With running, you're adding a new sport, new friends, and new experiences to your life.

done since the dawn of time. According to evolutionary biologists, the first humans were long-distance athletes, running across the grasslands, stalking dinner. Dinner being some form of lean meat. And there was no pull-in at the Dairy Queen for dessert afterward.

Dieting, at least among the masses, is a relatively recent phenomenon. Some 47 percent of Americans are trying to lose weight at any given time, according to the Centers for Disease Control and Prevention, or CDC. But when two out of every three adults in America are overweight, that's somewhat understandable.

So think of how you would rather lose weight and what you would like to tell people. What would you rather tell yourself? That you're learning a new sport? Or that you're on a diet?

WHAT THIS BOOK IS SELLING

RYBO is based on the understanding that in weight loss, there are no silver bullets or magic solutions. Losing weight requires work. If it weren't so challenging, America wouldn't be confronting the weight problem it faces today. First Lady Michelle Obama wouldn't have dedicated herself to the national crisis of childhood obesity through her "Let's Move" initiative.

The human body is highly adept at storing fat, and once it has fat, it guards it jealously. For most of human history, food was in short supply, so the body developed mechanisms to store extra energy in case of emergency. These days, we don't have to worry so much about days passing without nourishment, but our bodies still function as though we do. As a result, it takes a lot of effort to pry fat loose. We know it's not easy. Best to be honest about that.

SLOW, SLOW, SLOW

Losing weight is not effortless, nor is it quick. Let's go over how fast the weight should come off: The National Institutes of Health suggests trying to lose $\frac{1}{2}$ to 1 pound per week. On the low end, that works out to roughly

2 pounds per month, or about 12 to 17 pounds over the course of half a year. It may surprise you to learn what a slow process losing weight is. Remember this when you're setting expectations for yourself. And if you find a diet plan that promises faster weight loss, be careful about what you're getting yourself into, because you could be shedding water weight or muscle or using a program that is unsustainable. *RYBO* isn't a crash diet. Instead, it's an introduction to a new sport and a new way of thinking about food, which will lead to gradual, sustainable weight loss.

A SIMPLE MATH PROBLEM

While losing weight may require some effort, the math behind it is pretty easy. In order to shed pounds, you need to burn more calories, or take in fewer calories than your body uses in a day. Your goal is to create a calorie deficit.

There are three ways to go about creating this deficit.

1. You can eat less.

2. You can exercise more.

3. You can do both at the same time: Eat less and exercise more.

RYBO is focused on weight-loss strategy number three: Eat less while you exercise more.

Each of the following 10 chapters contains both an eating plan and an exercise plan, which will gradually take you from walking to running. Why running? Because we love it. It's fun to do. You don't need a gym or any specialized equipment that can be purchased only from an 800 number on an infomercial. It's affordable. All you really need is a decent pair of sneakers.

Want more reasons? You can run almost anywhere. Just park your car, get out, and go. In running, you burn more calories in less time than you do in almost any other sport. Plus, the postrun high, that feeling of well-being and accomplishment, is unrivaled. You just don't get the same feeling after you've stepped off a Stairmaster.

As mentioned earlier, we call the nutrition portion of *RYBO* an "eating plan," not a diet. Yes, you'll have to monitor the food you take in. A little bit of running is by no means permission to park yourself at the all-you-can-eat buffet. But think of this as a self-guided course in changing your eating habits and educating yourself. By doing some analysis of what you eat, when you eat, and how fast you gulp it down, you can pinpoint your dietary pitfalls—and learn how to avoid them. As you learn, you'll eat healthier (and less) without a constant, nagging, negative sense of self-denial.

HOW TO USE THIS BOOK

The workouts to get you to your weight-loss goals aren't supposed to be grueling. Far from it.

The aim of this book is to help you lose weight and become a runner.

This plan uses a gentle buildup. It starts with walking only, building up to 30 minutes at a time. The plan then includes some running. One minute at first. When you're ready, 2 minutes. Then 3, 5, 7 minutes. At a rate you determine, those 30 minutes of walking morph into 30 minutes of nonstop running.

The plan is presented in 12 stages. You can complete each stage in a week, so you could be finished in as few as 12 weeks. Or you can opt to take it much slower than that. Repeat each chapter's workout for 2 or even 3 weeks, if necessary. Stretch out the whole process to take 6 months or longer, if you feel more comfortable doing it that way.

In other words, take as long as you need to become a runner. We've found that although it may take some time, once you're a runner, you will want to stay a runner.

Consistency will help you get there. When you begin exercising, you need to stick with it, week in and week out. You need to find time to work out at least 3—preferably 4—days a week, and keep that appointment with yourself. The repetition is what makes running easier. With that dedication over a period of weeks and months, you'll strengthen your cardiovascular system, which is responsible for pumping oxygen to the muscles. (Some people call this getting into shape.) As you develop your heart and lungs, exercise feels better. And you'll be better able to nudge your body to relinquish its closely guarded fat.

YOUR UNIQUE CALCULATIONS

This book asks you to do some basic math to learn more about your body and the calories it needs in a day. Weight loss happens when you eat fewer calories and burn more, so you need to educate yourself about where you are now, how many calories you'll have to cut to lose weight, and how your new exercise program will add to that caloric deficit. Keep a calculator and a pencil handy. In a few spots, we'll ask you to access www.runnersworld. com for some specialized tools that compute calorie use and take gender, age, and activity level into account.

This is a learning process. To have success, you have to study this a little bit up front. Many people start exercising, breaking a sweat for the first time in years, and they're offended when the weight doesn't melt off as fast as they think it should. They fail to reckon with how their eating habits are affecting their caloric total for the day. With a little math, you'll have a lot more knowledge. And with knowledge, you'll see results.

A WORKBOOK TO MAKE IT EASY

We've developed a companion workbook, which you can find at the end of this book, to help you track your vital statistics: your weight each week, your calorie totals, and your workouts. With everything in one place, you'll be able to develop a plan for running and weight loss that makes sense for you. The workbook gives you a place to do the math this book asks for. No one has to see your personal data besides you, but we firmly believe that when you have those numbers in front of you, you'll be equipped to make better decisions about eating and exercise. Plus, there's

Meet Our Experts!

Now it's time to introduce the brains and bodies behind this book.

We have **Leslie Bonci**, MPH, RD, CSSD, LDN. Yep, she's earned a lot of degrees, but for our purposes she's director of sports nutrition at the University of Pittsburgh Medical Center. She helps everyone from individual clients struggling to lose weight to scholarship athletes at Pitt who need to eat for better performance. Most important, Leslie gets it. She runs 6 days a week, shops at a regular grocery store, and has raised two sons while working full-time. She understands the time and financial pressures we all face in our efforts to eat better.

The running plan comes from **Budd Coates**, who has a degree in exercise physiology and is senior director of health and fitness at Rodale Inc. (the company that publishes *Runner's World*), and an avid distance runner for 37 years. He competed in the US Olympic Marathon Trials four times, from 1984 to 1996, and he has a marathon personal best of 2:13. Budd has also worked with beginning runners for more than 30 years, encouraging them to take it easy, stick with it, and enjoy what running has to offer.

What beginners often don't know about Budd is that his father died of a heart attack at age 43. So Budd has always seen running as a lifestyle imperative that will protect his own ticker and keep his wife and kids from experiencing what he went through with the sudden loss of his dad.

As for me, I'm **Sarah Lorge Butler**. I'm a writer and I love running; I try to get out there four times a week. I've met some of my best friends through the sport, and I hope my daughter and son will grow up to share my feeling that a good run solves most of the stressful situations a person encounters in a day.

something satisfying about writing it down. It's always nice to put a checkmark next to a task you've accomplished.

REAL PEOPLE, REAL WEIGHT LOSS

We also assembled a test panel to try out our plan. We found 16 good-natured women and men who wanted to lose weight and were willing to give running—and eating better—a try. Most of them had been struggling with the number on the scale for years; many had tried multiple diets. They range in age from 24 to 57 and have all kinds of jobs and dozens of kids between them. They're real people who have been around the block, literally and figuratively.

First they walked, then they ran. Many are now running farther than they ever thought possible. Fourteen of them lost weight during our 12-week test, somewhere between 8 and 26 pounds. One stayed exactly the same. And one gained 2 pounds (though she was the lowest weight to begin with, and she lost nearly 2 inches from her waist). This is real life, folks.

While they were at it, our test panelists showered Leslie, Budd, and me with honest feedback about their triumphs, their struggles, the changes that were easy to make, and those that were more difficult to incorporate. Enjoy their reflections. You might just recognize yourself in them.

The test panel also gives us vivid examples of how weight loss happens differently for different people. Julie, a 38-year-old, started at 184 pounds and lost 13, even losing during those busy weeks when she couldn't fit in all her scheduled workouts. Same for Dorene, a former physical education teacher who quickly lost 16 pounds. Her training partner, Stephanie, who ran every step alongside Dorene, lost steadily between ½ and 1 pound a week for 7 weeks, then hit a plateau for 2 weeks.

It's frustrating when the woman next to you, doing exactly the same exercise and eating just about the same foods, is losing faster than you are. Scientists, doctors, and dietitians could theorize endlessly about why this is so. Genetics, body composition, and other daily activity all play a role. But the annoying reality remains: Weight comes off faster for some than it does for others.

All of this is a way of saying that you have to celebrate the successes, roll with the setbacks, and be happy with what you're doing for yourself. If you follow this book to the end, we're certain you'll lose some weight. And we can guarantee you'll be better off than when you started. Because you'll have a new sport. You'll be a runner.

Chapter 1

Get Moving!

Forget what you've watched on *The Biggest Loser*. We're not sending you out for a 2-hour workout on your first day. Sorry if that news comes as a disappointment.

This program isn't boot camp, and it isn't punishment. The last thing we want is for you to get discouraged during the first week.

We start slowly and build slowly and run slowly. The weight might come off more gradually than if you took on a crash program, but doing it this way, the pounds are more likely to stay off. And you'll be a heck of a lot healthier in the long run by finding a routine you can stick with.

> We start slowly and build slowly and run slowly.

That said, you have homework to do this week, but it's not the physical kind. If you're going to do this right, the program requires some preparation—self-guided study, if you will. And you've got to get ready for running.

We'll get you out the door for your first workout in a few moments, but stick with us here as we go over some basics.

FINDING THE TIME

When you're introducing formal, regular exercise into your schedule, you need to build it into your day as if it were any other appointment, like a dentist visit or a parent-teacher conference, only more enjoyable. (Maybe like a haircut or coffee with friends?) You don't blow off going to work every morning, nor should you skip your exercise appointment. If you don't organize an exercise timetable and instead leave it to chance, trust us when we say: Your workout is not going to happen.

It took me 5 years of parenthood to learn this lesson. Countless times I'd go to bed at night thinking I'd run in the morning. My alarm would go off and I'd hit "snooze," rationalizing to myself that I'd exercise when my husband got home from work. Inevitably, either he'd be held up at the office or I'd be preparing dinner when he walked in, and my motivation to exercise was greatly diminished when I considered the alternative of sitting down to a meal with my family.

Last winter we took a new approach: Sunday evenings, we'd get out our calendars and plan our workouts—my running and swimming, his tennis. I'd set out my clothes or gym bag the night before I was supposed to get up early. We'd leave the car outside so the sound of the garage door under the kids' bedrooms didn't wake them up early. Every time, within 90 seconds of getting out of bed, I was glad I had. It felt great to get one thing checked off my to-do list before 7:00 a.m., and I've drastically decreased the number of evenings when I've been annoyed with myself for skipping exercise that day.

Which isn't to say your exercise has to happen in the morning. It just has to happen 30 minutes four times a week. This is no mean feat. The time pressures we face are incredible. Most of us are putting in at least an 8-hour workday, not including commuting time. When we're home we have children to look after, and if they're young, there are endless trips driving them to dance and soccer and T-ball. Or we need to look in on our parents or be available to take an after-hours work call from Asia. It's nuts.

People manage to exercise, though. Over the years, *Runner's World* editors have heard from folks who get awfully creative about squeezing in their workouts. One guy we talked to runs laps around his kids' soccer practice. A consultant told us he has mapped out running routes from all his clients' offices and hits the road immediately after meetings, changing

---

Budd's Buzz: "My son is a competitive gymnast, and for years I've been driving him to practice in the afternoons, dropping him off, then going for a run. Most of the parents sit in the bleachers to watch. I usually return about 10 minutes before practice ends, and almost every time one of the other parents will say to me, 'Oh, you're a runner? I wish I had time to run.' That drives me crazy! If you've been sitting here for an hour, you have time to run!"

---

in his car and washing off his sweat with special wipes, Nathan's Power Shower. One woman runs to the daycare center after work to pick up her daughter, and her husband meets them there and drives them home.

Other folks are squeezing in time at lunch, working through lunch 3 days a week and extending their lunch hours on the other 2 days to run and shower. Some folks have wised up enough to change into their workout gear at the office and go straight to the park before going home, because once you actually get those sneakers on, exercise seems more doable. Wait until you get home? Forget it. Someone always needs you. Or the couch beckons.

SCHEDULE THE APPOINTMENT

Please learn from my 5 years of frustration: Get your calendar (whatever form it takes) and figure out when you can find 30 minutes of time for uninterrupted exercise at least four times a week. You can also use the companion personal workbook at the end of this book to schedule your workouts. If you have to enlist a grandparent or a babysitter to watch the kids for the 45 minutes you'll need for exercise and a shower, I'm a fan of that strategy.

When we say "uninterrupted," we mean it's best to leave the dog or the baby jogger at home, especially when you're getting used to this new routine. Maybe your kids will fall asleep in a jogger, but mine were always good for about 12 minutes before they started fretting. I'd be tossing bits of bagel down at them to keep them occupied, pleading, "Oh, just 5 more minutes. Honey, look at the squirrel!" Eventually I'd give up. Another day, another partial workout. And while a partial workout is better than no workout, it's preferable to carve out an uninterrupted block of time, especially while you're getting used to integrating exercise into your life.

THE MAGIC OF FOUR

Do you need 4 days? Well, truth be told, 3 are okay, especially if you're exercising for the first time. But you'll see results so much faster if you can fit in four sessions. You'll be boosting your calorie burn over the course of the week with that extra session. And in less time you'll start feeling better (breathing easier, moving easier, sleeping sounder). Best to schedule 4 days, with the understanding that if something unexpected crops up in your week, you have a 1-day cushion.

BE STUBBORN!

Protect your exercise time! Guard it. You are *so worth* the 2 hours per week. Many of us devote time to taking care of other people—kids, spouses, elderly parents, demanding bosses. It's time to do something for *you*.

> Protect your exercise time! You are *so worth* the 2 hours per week.

While you're scheduling, it's best to give yourself a break between days when possible, rather than going 4 in a row and 3 off. An off day in between has both physical and mental benefits. Obviously, if you're going to exercise on 4 out of 7 days in a week, you'll need to go back-to-back at least once. But space it as best you can. Monday, Wednesday, Friday, Saturday is a popular plan. Or Tuesday, Thursday, Saturday, Sunday, which allows you to make use of both weekend days.

The point is this: Come up with a schedule you can live with. This is the key to your success with *RYOB*.

Budd's Buzz: "The biggest thing is looking long-term. Develop consistency in your new lifestyle. The mistake people make is that they try to do a whole lot all at once, and then they take a period of time off. Then they do that again: a whole lot at once, followed by a long time off. When you're putting together the schedule, ask yourself, *Can I do this over and over?*"

Our test panel was made up of plenty of busy folks. And then there's Amy W. She's a 34-year-old mother of two little ones. She works full-time as an admissions officer for a college. On weekends she's involved with her church and shuttling her kids to their activities. And she has battled cancer: She beat stage IV lymphoma in 2008 and got through a bout with thyroid cancer in 2009. She's one tough cookie.

If anyone has an excuse to sleep in, it's Amy. Here's what a typical week looks like for her, in her own words.

6:00 a.m.:	Wake up to run. (Monday and Wednesday; Saturdays I run a little later.)
6:30 a.m.:	Wake up all other days.
7:00 to 7:30 a.m.:	Get kids and myself ready. My husband helps a lot with the kids in the morning and takes them to school.
8:00 a.m.:	Arrive at work.
Lunch:	Work out in my office with a toning video that uses weights and a stability ball—either Monday, Wednesday, and Friday or Tuesday and Thursday, depending on the week.
4:30ish:	Leave work and pick up the kids 20 minutes away. Thursday nights I work until 5:55 and then meet the running group at 6:00.
5:00 to 8:30 p.m.:	Variety of evening activities with the kids, including swimming, going to the park, playing in the backyard, going for a walk, homework, dinner, dishes, soccer practice, shopping, keeping up with housework, bath time, preparing lunches for the next day, and bedtime for the kids.

8:30 to 9:30 p.m.: Finish up anything I didn't get done between 5 and 8:30.

9:30 to 10:00 p.m.: Wind down with a little TV, then read or play brain games on my DS before bed.

10 p.m.: Lights out. I try to go to bed around 10:00 so that I can get up and run the next day.

Let's see. Amy gets four runs in: Monday and Wednesday morning, Thursday evening with a running group, and Saturday morning with her best friend from high school. She also manages to do the 20-minute Denise Austin toning video in the middle of her workday two or three times a week. And what she fails to mention here is that she still has to work in countless doctors' appointments for herself, including periodic 5-hour maintenance treatments to counter the lymphoma.

Looking at that week is a huge motivation for me. Maybe you'll agree with my assessment: If Amy can find 2 hours for four running workouts each week while fighting cancer, I can certainly find the time.

LOCATION, LOCATION, LOCATION

Do some poking around for a good spot to begin your walking. Eventually the walking evolves into running, so the location is important. It's great if you live in a neighborhood where you can start moving straight from your front door, but that's not always feasible.

If you have to commute to your workout, look for parks that have walking or biking trails. Packed-down dirt-cinder paths are ideal because that softer surface is forgiving on your feet, ankles, shins, and knees, but a paved path will do nicely. Either way, you don't have to stop for traffic, and if you're lucky, you'll have access to bathrooms and drinking fountains. Don't have anything like that where you live? Then look for a route with few traffic lights, so you don't have to stop while you're waiting for the light to change. Low traffic volume and wide shoulders on the road are big pluses, too.

(continued on page 10)

What Should I Wear?

When you first start to run, you have enough things to worry about: your breathing, your legs, and that nagging feeling that everyone is looking at you, passing judgment. The last thing you want to think about is your clothing. You need your outfits to make you comfortable, not more self-conscious.

The best clothes for beginning runners are the pieces you don't notice. They fit the right way; don't ride up, bunch, or chafe; and they flatter the figure. It takes a little trial and error to find that gear.

Apparel manufacturers try to convince us that we need expensive, high-tech fabrics that keep sweat away from the body. That's known as "moisture wicking" in marketing parlance. Some test panelists swear by these "technical" shirts and shorts. Others stick to the comfy cotton tees they've worn for years. Stores like Target or Kohl's carry moisture-wicking clothes at a lower cost, so you don't have to spend a lot to see if you like them.

When the test panelists found running outfits they liked, they became very loyal to those brands. Their responses to the question "What should a beginning runner wear?" yielded a variety of suggestions at a wide range of price points to accommodate runners of all sizes. Here's a head-to-toe guide to feeling comfortable on the run.

Headwear: Some runners wear hats or visors for every workout; other runners feel like headwear is a distraction that only makes them sweat more. If you run outdoors in the middle of the day, a hat will provide protection from the sun. For nighttime runs, a hat with reflective stripes can make you more visible to traffic.

Bras: A good sports bra for women is a must-have. "My local running store has Bra Fest once a summer," test panelist Amy N. says. "They set out wine and cheese, and the Moving Comfort ladies bring all their bra styles in every single size they carry, and they'll find you a perfect fit."

Tops: At the beginning runner level, wear whatever feels comfortable. Cotton retains moisture, but assuming you're running for only 30 to 45 minutes and you're not climbing Mount Everest later in the day, a damp tee isn't a problem. Others swear by technical tops, which keep them from getting too sweaty and clammy. Look for a generous fit around the underarms, which can be a common spot for chafing.

Bottoms: Test panelists say longer is better as you start out. Many opt for Capri-length pants or knee-length spandex, because shorter running shorts can chafe between the thighs. "I found that shorter shorts worked their way up, and I was constantly pulling them down between my thighs," says Donna. "Once I started losing weight in my thighs, shorter shorts became more comfortable." A pocket for car keys is a plus.

Socks: Again, the debate here is cotton versus technical. And while a wet top won't be too problematic, when your feet sweat, you're more prone to blisters.

Shoes: Be sure to go to a specialty running store and ask for your feet to be measured. Our feet change through the decades; two test panelists discovered they had been wearing running sneakers that were too small.

Scope out a route that's relatively flat. When you're getting used to walking and running, it can feel like a major effort to your lungs. Big hills will only intensify that feeling of work. Remember, we're trying to take small steps here. You can add the hills when you're a little more experienced.

Tracks can be a good choice if you don't get bored going around in a circle. They're flat, obviously, and the rubberized surface is gentler on your legs than the road is. If you're curious about the distance you've gone, you can keep track of your laps. Here's a hint: If you use a track, stick to the outside lanes until you're a much more experienced runner. Lanes one and two are for those racers who are trying to do high-speed intervals and shave a few seconds off their next race. You don't want to get run over.

When you have your exercise appointments scheduled and you've found a good place, you're ready to go. This program starts with walking. Before you can try running, you need to be able to complete four walks, each one 30 minutes nonstop, in a week.

STAGE 1 WORKOUT

• Walk for 30 minutes.

Total workout time: 30 minutes.

Do this workout at least three or four times in a week
before moving on to the next stage.

You might be able to do that this week without a problem. In that case, once you've done four walking workouts, you're ready to proceed to the next stage.

Or you might need to start at less than 30 minutes, depending on what kind of shape you're in and how much extra weight you're carrying around.

What kind of pace should you walk at? Pick something that's comfortable—steady, not aggressive. Aim for a pace that's a little faster than your stroll-down-the-driveway-in-your-slippers-to-get-the-newspaper walk but slower than your might-miss-my-connecting-flight walk. Don't sweat the pace, just get out and do it.

You do not want to be huffing and puffing. If you're panting, you're going too fast. Remember, this isn't punitive. You're not supposed to finish each workout feeling like you need a nap.

In the weeks ahead, as you start to integrate running segments into the workout, walking is going to be the recovery portion, the time when you take it easy and catch your breath. So if walking has you breathing heavy, it's too fast. Slow it down.

Your breathing is an instantaneous check of your effort level. Take the "talk test." If you can get a few sentences out, you're fine. If you need to pause for a breath between words, take your foot off the gas until you can talk comfortably.

THE POWER OF WALKING

Why do we like walking so much? Walking is fantastic exercise. You can do it anywhere. It's great for your heart and lungs. And, most important for *RYBO,* walking gets you ready to run.

In walking, you're doing almost exactly the same thing you do when you run, except one foot is on the ground at all times. But you build the same leg muscles, which you'll need to propel yourself forward when you do start to run. You also build bone density and strengthen the ligaments and tendons in the joints in your legs. It's good stuff.

The cardiovascular benefits are similar to those running provides. When you first get used to regular walking, you're conditioning your heart to be better at pumping oxygen to your muscles. And walking burns calories. I know that if I sit on the couch for 30 minutes, I burn about 28 calories. If I walk for 30 minutes, about 1½ miles, I burn 103 calories. When weight loss is your goal, walking contributes to that almighty deficit you're trying to create.

> Have faith, and a little patience. Walk before you run.

A warning to you former runners: You're not exempt from this step. Yeah, you, the one who ran the 800 meters on the high school track team 25 years ago. We know what's going through your head: *Walking is for wimps. If I'm going to get back into shape,* you're thinking, *I'm going to run. I can skip this chapter.*

Not so fast. Why rush it? Walking is easier on the legs and back than running is, so use it to shed your first few pounds, get back into a routine, and then start jogging again. If you go straight to running with an extra

 FOOD TALK ## A Little Background

Here's what we know: A pound of fat is equivalent to about 3,500 calories. Consume 3,500 more than your body can use, and you'll gain a pound. That's the calculation the media use when you see those headlines: "Extra! Extra! If You Overeat by 100 Calories a Day, You'll Gain 10 Pounds a Year!" (That's correct, by the way.)

But right now there's one great unknown. You don't know how many calories your body needs in a day.

SECRETS OF THE TEST PANEL

AMY W., 34

Job: College admissions counselor; mother of two

Goals: Lose 20 pounds and be able to run a 5-K

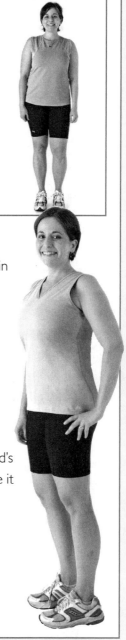

Starting weight: 163 pounds

Ending Weight: 155 pounds

Starting waist: 37 inches

Ending waist: 34 inches

"Wow!" Moment: I can run a mile in a little more than 10 minutes now—comfortably! I talk about running a lot, and that's helped me recruit two new friends to run with. I finished a 5-K in 36:20, and that included a 2-minute walk.

Secret Weapon: Friends! Running with friends makes it so much easier. We're all so busy that it's the only time we have to chat without kids.

No Excuses: I have come to the conclusion that I have the power to make the change. It's my fault if I don't reach my goals—not my kids' fault or my husband's fault. I am the one in control, and it's up to me to make it work.

10, 20, or 30 pounds, that's a lot more force you'll be putting on your joints. Have faith, and a little patience. Walk before you run. Walking is excellent for all the reasons we've talked about. It's not for wusses.

HOW MANY CALORIES DO YOU NEED?

As we mentioned previously, it's worth doing a little homework along with this program. In making some preliminary calculations about the calories your body uses in a day, you get a much more accurate picture of what you need to do to lose weight. You'll have a lot more success with this program if you're not flying blind. So get ready.

A little good news: Your body burns calories all the time, even when you're sitting on the couch watching *Oprah*. When you're commenting on friends' status on Facebook. Even when you're sleeping. The body needs energy for all of its functions—for breathing, for your heart to beat, and for your blood to circulate.

This basic rate of calorie burn—what you burn when you're at rest—is called your basal metabolic rate, or BMR for short. Everyone has a different BMR. The number changes depending on how big you are to start with and how much of your size is muscle or fat.

So how can you figure out your own magic number? Well, different formulas exist for calculating it. The most accurate measures rely on sophisticated body composition analysis. We assume you don't have access to that kind of testing right now. Thankfully, there are many online resources that will give you a pretty close idea—close enough so that you can be informed about what you need to do to lose weight.

Don't sweat this. These calculators want only four variables: your weight, height, gender, and age. I entered my measurements in a variety of calculators, and they all spit back at me a BMR number within 15 calories of each other.

We've built one you can use at: runnersworld.com/rybo.

We'll pause while you go to your computer and figure yours out. You can enter your number, in pencil, below.

My BMR: _____

A little good news: Your body burns calories all the time.

Congratulations! You've calculated your first BMR.

We'll also direct you to enter this number in the back now, in the Personal Workbook Week 1, so you have all your important numbers in one place. We've also included the equations there for your reference.

Why in pencil? Well, this piece of news may be a bit of a bummer: As you lose weight, your BMR—the number of calories you need in a day to function at rest—goes down, too. Five pounds might not affect it significantly, but if you find yourself losing 10, 20, or 30 pounds, as we hope, that BMR number starts to take a dive. Sorry to have to break that to you. We'll remind you to recalculate toward the end of the book.

Now you understand the number of calories your body uses at rest, your BMR.

My BMR is 1,362. That's the number of calories I burn when vegging out, doing absolutely nothing. That's 56 calories per hour. Honestly, that doesn't seem like very many, especially when I consider that six peanut M&M's have about 60 calories.

Of course, few of us are truly that sedentary. We're doing some moving. We're walking around the house, climbing stairs, standing in line at the post office, lifting kids in and out of their car seats, pushing a cart through a grocery store, unloading the groceries and putting them away, folding laundry. And maybe your job requires some standing and walking around. If you're a teacher, you're striding the halls of a school, or if you're a nurse at a hospital, you're constantly on your feet. Some people have truly physical jobs, like highway road crews, roofers, and landscapers dragging tree branches out of the way.

So you get to add a little bit to your BMR. Because, of course, any physical activity beyond what you burn lying in bed requires extra calories.

How much? Here, Budd and Leslie like the Harris-Benedict equation, which was developed by scientists in Boston in the early part of the 20th century and is still widely accepted today. Once you get your BMR, you multiply it by a factor ranging from 1.2 (sedentary) to 1.9 (lumberjack), depending on how much activity you get during the day. There are five activity levels on the scale, and you can do the multiplication here: www.runnersworld.com/rybo.

- If you are sedentary, multiply your BMR × 1.2.
- If you are lightly active, multiply your BMR × 1.375.
- If you are moderately active, multiply your BMR × 1.55.
- If you are very active, multiply your BMR × 1.725.
- If you are extra active, multiply your BMR × 1.9.

For the purposes of *RYBO,* pick an activity level that matches your movement before you do any organized, purposeful exercise. I figure that, without my running, I'm lightly active, especially in the winter. In the summer maybe I'm a little more active, spending more time at the park and in the pool. But to err on the side of realism, I'm going to use the lightly active factor, 1.375. Multiply that by my BMR (1,362) and voilà— I need about 1,873 calories to get through the day at my current activity level, before I add in my running.

Go ahead, do the calculation. Take the BMR you discovered on page 15, multiply it by one of the Harris-Benedict factors, and enter it here.

My total calorie needs: _____

This is the number of calories you need to maintain your current weight. Ideally, you should be eating about that number every day. If you eat more than your total calorie needs, you're gaining weight. It may be a slow creep, but you're gaining. You have to get to neutral before you can start to think about losing.

We give you this number as a baseline. The purpose of this number is to give you a realistic view of how certain foods and habits can sabotage or enhance an eating plan. Ripping into a can of Pringles at night, even if everything else you've eaten has been healthy, can greatly affect your total for the day. Substituting fruits and veggies with yogurt for a New York–style bagel can send the number the other way. But think of this in broad terms. Don't drive yourself crazy with calculating calories to the decimal point.

The number also shows you the role exercise plays in weight loss. Jacking up the burn consistently over time can help create that all-important deficit you need for fat loss. You should be starting to see, on an intellectual level at least, how you can change these numbers to create a deficit.

> If you eat more than your total calorie needs, you're gaining weight.

The next step is actually creating that deficit, not on an intellectual level, but on a kitchen cupboard and running shoes level. That's what we'll show you how to do in the upcoming chapters.

JENNIFER, 27

Job: Scientist

Goals: Lose weight, become healthier, and stick
with it

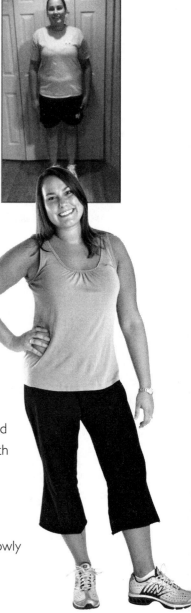

Starting weight: 212 pounds

Ending weight: 190 pounds

How I Got Here: Right after college, I started a
job as a lab tech and was commuting 45 minutes
each way. Then I got promoted to supervisor, and
it was my job to get things done on a deadline. I
would end up working through lunch and then
staying 2 or 3 hours late at night. By the time I
got home, either I was not hungry at all and
completely skipped dinner or I was starving
and I'd stop on the way back for fast food.
And then I'd get home and plop—I wouldn't
want to do anything.

A Former Athlete: I was a competitive swimmer
in high school and college, so I thought everything had
to be fast. If I started running and I'd get out of breath
quickly, I'd lose my motivation. Or I'd start other
exercise plans, then give up after a few sessions of
overdoing it without really seeing results.

Secret Weapon: The treadmill. Learning to run slowly

has been so important for me. I like the treadmill because I can keep it at a steady speed. Even now when I run outside, I'll notice that I start running too fast and I'm tired 15 or 20 minutes in. And it helps to listen to whatever I want on my iPod, usually horrible eighties music. When I'm on the treadmill by myself, I catch myself either singing along or "dance walking" after a run. It's a good thing they make that safety cord that turns off the belt, as I have had a few close calls with overeager dance walking!

Slow Buildup: The running plan is great because it's so gradual. A lot of my friends thought I just started running 3 miles at a time, but that simply isn't feasible if you're carrying extra weight.

No Excuses: Every once in a while I do have to talk myself into running, but then again, it's only a 30-minute workout. To find a half-decent excuse would take 15 minutes, so at that point I might as well have just started running.

Plan Ahead: I try to take a few minutes to sit down and eat. I started buying portable, healthier foods to munch on in the car when I really don't have the time. The planning is helpful. I may not be really hungry right at that moment, but I know I do need to eat something instead of skipping a meal and eating a ton of food later.

Skip the Scale: I don't weigh myself too often—every other week or so. My pants are a better guide. When I started the program, my pants got so loose, I had to buy a few new pairs in quick succession.

Chapter 2

"If I have the belief that I can do it, I shall surely acquire the capacity to do it even if I may not have it at the beginning."
—*Mahatma Gandhi*

It Starts with a Single Step

The pages of *Runner's World* are filled with famous writers singing the praises of running. We think it's pretty cool, too. When running feels good, it feels great.

Of course, when you're just starting, it feels hard. Damn hard. Exhausting even. It's work. A runner's high? You gotta be kidding me.

We hear you. All runners, even the most experienced ones, have days when their legs feel like cinder blocks, or their lungs feel hopelessly inadequate. Their panting is worse than a dog's on a summer day. And that's before the chafing.

When you're heavier than you want to be and you haven't been active in a long time, it really is difficult, both physically and mentally, to start running. We understand that. It takes a lot of courage to even try. Those first few steps are a leap of faith, and we give you so much credit for giving it a shot.

Stick with us long enough, though, and one day you will feel the great side of it. You'll be out there and you'll have a buddy alongside you, cracking you up with his latest stories. Before you realize it, a mile will have gone by, and then another. You won't believe how effortless it feels. Later on you'll glance in the mirror as you're coming out of the shower and you'll think, *My calves look pretty cut, if I do say so myself.* Or you'll notice how with a postrun flush your face looks better than anything you could get from the Clinique counter. After a good run, there's a sense of calm that stays with you through your day and defuses all your interactions with potentially difficult people: your kids, your coworkers, your mother-in-law.

That running nirvana, most likely, is several weeks or months off in your future.

> Those first few steps are a leap of faith.

For now it's going to feel like a major effort. But even while you're exerting yourself, know what you're doing: Your heart is getting stronger, your lungs are breathing deeper. The results aren't just on the scale.

You may see your blood pressure, cholesterol, and triglycerides drop. Dorene on our test panel watched her blood pressure go from 140/90 in the first week of the study to 118/78 by the end. Her LDL ("bad") cholesterol and triglycerides dropped 20 points each. Her doctor even reduced the dosage of her thyroid medication.

You're building muscles everywhere, especially in your legs, but also in your core due to all your deep breathing. You're increasing bone density. Then there are the "soft" benefits: the calm, the sense of achievement, the sounder sleep at night.

 ## Why Running?

Why does running give you so much more bang for your exercise buck? It's partly a matter of physics. When you walk, you always have one foot on the ground. When you run, you get momentarily airborne. Amby Burfoot, editor at large of *Runner's World* and the 1968 Boston Marathon champion, put it this way in a 2004 article about weight loss:

> Running and walking aren't as comparable as I had imagined. When you walk, you keep your legs mostly straight, and your center of gravity rides along fairly smoothly on top of your legs. In running, we actually jump from one foot to the other. Each jump raises our center of gravity when we take off and lowers it when we land, since we bend the knee to absorb the shock. This continual rise and fall of our weight requires a tremendous amount of Newtonian force (fighting gravity) on both takeoff and landing.

So that's the "why" of running—and why we think it's a great plan for weight loss.

And here's the big one: When it comes to torching calories, nothing beats running. If a 200-pound person walks a mile, he or she will burn about 106 calories. Run the same mile, and the burn is about 150. Plus, as you become more experienced, you naturally get a little faster when you're running, so you get more done in less time. Other sports can't keep up with running's burn, and neither can ellipticals and stairclimbers. According to the Mayo Clinic, jogging trumps swimming, cycling, weight lifting, and aerobics in terms of calorie expenditure.

So yes, months down the road, as you develop into a runner, you can look forward to new worlds: new parks, new trails, new friends, and new races if you choose to enter them.

Short term, you'll enjoy losing weight at a faster clip.

Let's get to it.

STAGE 2 WORKOUT

- Walk for 4 minutes. Run for 1 minute.

- Repeat that sequence four more times.

- End with 4 minutes of walking.

Total workout time: 29 minutes, 5 of which are running.

Do this workout at least three or four times in a week
before moving on to the next stage.

Now you know what the second workout is. But before you rush out and try it, a few guidelines.

As you're starting out, you need to run slowly. Very slowly.

This is crucial, so I'll say it again.

As you're starting out, **YOU NEED TO RUN SLOWLY.** Very slowly.

How slow is slow? Try this: Make your run no faster than your walk. Yes, that's right: no faster than your walk. At this point, you have to set aside any preconceived notions you have about running. If the Presidential Physical Fitness testing of your youth still haunts you, fear not. No one is standing by you with a stopwatch. This run does not have to be fast, nor should it be. In these 1-minute running segments, you're not required to cover a set distance.

You simply have to get running, so your body is airborne between footfalls. If you did the Stage 1 workout, 30 minutes of nonstop walking, this small amount of running should not feel that much harder.

Just in case we didn't make it clear, we'll say it one more time:

As you're starting out, you need to run slowly. Very slowly.

> As you're starting out,
> YOU NEED TO RUN
> SLOWLY.

A new runner I know, Barbara, discovered this strategy of slow running on her own. In November 2009, she was 48 years old, and she wanted to lose 25 to 30 pounds.

An assistant general manager for a software company, Barbara was working between 60 and 80 hours per week. She was getting up at 5:00 a.m. every day, checking in with her team in India, and if all was well, she would start her workout. She had a treadmill in her basement, and she worked up to 30 minutes of walking on it at a brisk pace, about 4.5 miles per hour. She wanted to get more out of her 30 minutes of cardio, so she decided to try running.

But she had a fear about running. "I had visions I'd go flying off the back of the treadmill and crash through the wall behind me," she said. So

---

Budd's Buzz: "Try to keep your breathing under control. If you're looking at your watch and you're thinking, *When will this minute be over?* you're going too fast."

she actually reduced the speed on the treadmill, back to 3.5 mph, for her first few attempts at running. Her thought was that if she felt out of control, she could always stop and walk, and she already knew she could walk at 3.5 mph. At first she ran at 3.5 mph for 30 seconds. Then the next day she tried a minute. Then she ran until the end of a good song playing on her iPod. Nothing catastrophic happened. She didn't slam into any walls.

Well, you can probably guess where this story goes. Soon Barbara moved the speed up to 3.6 mph, then 3.7. Within about 3 weeks, she could run a mile without stopping. A month later, she was running for 30 minutes straight on the treadmill. Then came the races: a 5-K followed by a couple of 5-milers. When she turned 50, she signed up for a half-marathon.

In April 2010, Barbara finished her first half-marathon in 2 hours 27 minutes. She was ecstatic. Oh, and those 25 pounds she wanted to shed? She lost 40. It all started with a 30-second run on her treadmill at slower than her walking pace.

That can be you, too. Start off as if you were going on any old 30-minute walk, like you have been for at least the past week. After the first 4 minutes of walking, try running. Think of it as picking up your feet, not picking up the pace. You don't need to cover a whole lot of extra ground. Return to your walking pace. See how this feels.

 # A Word on Shoes

At this point, do you need to rush out and buy new running shoes? No. Your cross-trainers are probably fine. Remember, you're running only 20 minutes a week in this stage. Next stage you'll do 40 minutes a week. If you really, really, really want to buy yourself new running shoes, go for it. But unless you want to drop $100 or more right now, you can probably wait until Stage 5. We'll revisit the topic then.

A STOPWATCH IS A GOOD IDEA

While you probably can get by with the sneakers you have, a stopwatch comes in mighty handy. This is a digital watch that might include alarms and timers, but all you need is the stopwatch function. The digital display shows you in minutes and seconds how long you've been moving. Because you're slowly increasing the running interval by a minute at a time, it's best to have one of these suckers. You don't have to buy a fancy GPS watch, like a Garmin. Try something no-frills, like a Timex. Search Amazon.com for "Timex Sports Watch" and you'll find them as cheap as $15. Walmart and Target also carry inexpensive stopwatches. Believe me, they make keeping track of your workouts much easier.

BRACE YOURSELF: MORE MATH ON THE WAY!

Back to the point about creating a calorie deficit. That's why we're here, after all. As we discussed in the first chapter, a pound of fat is about 3,500 calories. So to lose a pound a week, which is the upper end of the range of what the National Institutes of Health says is reasonable, you have to create a caloric deficit of about 500 calories per day.

In Chapter 1, you calculated your total daily calorie needs, without including formal exercise sessions. Remember: To lose weight, you have three choices. You can eat less than your body needs, burn more than you typically burn, or do both: Eat less and burn more.

So what kind of calories does this workout use? It's hard to know exactly, because it does depend somewhat on your intensity. One person might cover 2 miles with this workout. Another might make it only 1½ miles. But we can give you an estimate based on a 2004 study by researchers at Syracuse University called "Energy Expenditure of Walking and Running." Take your body weight in pounds and multiply it by 0.53, and that gives you the calories you burn walking 1 mile. For running, you can use 0.75 times your weight in pounds to give you calories used.

Let's imagine you weigh 200 pounds. And in the Stage 2 workout, let's assume you're able to cover 1.7 miles, most of it walking. Because there's so little running at first, we'll use the walking factor: 0.53 (walking calories burned per mile) × 200 pounds (body weight in pounds) = 106 calories burned per mile. Multiply that by the total distance, 1.7 miles, and you get 180 calories. (A 160-pound person would have burned 144 calories. That's because the more you weigh, the more effort it takes to move your mass and the more calories you burn.) Bear in mind that this is an estimate, because we don't know the exact distance covered.

At the end of this chapter, check out the chart where we've done some math for you to show how many calories you'll burn walking and running different distances.

But for now, let's say you, a 200-pound person, have burned about 180 calories. Does that seem like a lot?

Didn't think so.

It's kind of sobering to think that in the 60 seconds or so it takes you to eat a Dunkin' Donuts glazed doughnut, you can completely restore the calories you burned (and then some) during that 29-minute workout.

But it's good that you know it. First, that knowledge will give you motivation to stay away from the doughnuts. Second, you can be realistic about what you need to do to lose weight. Third, you realize the fallacy in thinking that because you're exercising, you can be free to eat anything you want.

And hey, don't be so glum. Multiply that 180 calories by 4, because you're doing four of those workouts a week, and you see you burn 720 calories. Now that is a reason to pat yourself on the back.

Now is a good time to talk about expectations. If, as experts say, reasonable weight loss is ½ to 1 pound per week, that works out to somewhere between 2 and 4 pounds per month. Great if it falls off faster, but if it doesn't, that's okay, too. Leslie and Budd both have witnessed folks losing a lot of weight quickly—then gaining it back even faster. Stick to the slow and steady and you'll be more likely to keep it off.

> Reasonable weight loss is ½ to 1 pound per week. That works out to somewhere between 2 and 4 pounds per month.

Again, to lose a pound a week, you need to create a deficit of about 500 calories per day. If you're okay with losing ½ pound a week, you'll need a deficit only half that size, or 250 calories per day, which works out to 1,750 calories per week. And when you estimate the exercise you're doing, this chapter's workout cuts anywhere from 500 to 750 calories a week, you're a good bit of the way there.

At the beginning, when you're mostly walking, exercise is a relatively small proportion of the calorie deficit you create. Stick with it, though. As you go through the program and gradually start running more, you'll burn more and more with each workout.

Leslie's Lessons: "Exercise is vitally important for so many health reasons, as well as to help with weight loss and successfully keep the weight off. But in the beginning especially, exercise is not the big-ticket item in terms of weight loss. It's the supporting role. Diet is the main character here. Exercise is occurring in one bout during the day. You have a chance to wheel and deal with your eating every time you eat."

Realize, though, that early on the best way for you to create that calorie deficit is by changing your eating habits. Which, by the way, does not excuse you from exercising!

Think of a calorie-burn-o-meter. Week 1, the needle is pointing mostly at the eating side. By Week 6, it might be in the middle. And by Week 10, it might be pointing over in the running side of things.

Where the calorie deficit comes from:

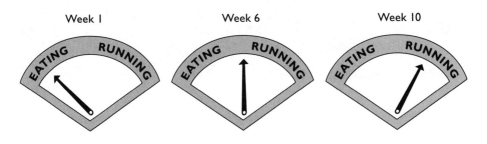

Week 1   Week 6   Week 10

FOOD TALK

Log It!

If you try to lose weight without examining your eating habits, it's like trying to hit a baseball with your eyes closed. Let's take an honest look at the state of your plate.

We're asking you to write down everything you eat for the next week. Every crust of your child's PB&J that finds its way into your mouth, every beer, every pretzel. Please, write it down. At the end of this book, you'll find a RYBO Food Log you can use for this purpose.

THE ALL-IMPORTANT FOOD LOG

The food log is asking for the when, what, where, why, and how much. You're a detective, and you're digging for the facts of your eating. You'll be amazed at what you find.

The first column asks for the time of day. Easy enough: Note the time.

Second, record where you are when you eat: at the kitchen table, dining room table, in the car, at your desk, or anywhere else.

The third one requires more detail: what you're eating. If it's soup, what kind? Cereal, what brand? Sandwich, what's on it? If you don't usually hold the mayo, then don't withhold it from your log, either.

The fourth column asks how much. It can be a challenge to know exactly how much pasta or cereal you ate or how many grapes you popped into your mouth. But give it a try.

The fifth column is an easy one. Put a notation for "H" if you were hungry when you ate, "NH" if you weren't hungry. If it's the latter, you were probably bored or overwhelmed or just wanted to crunch on something in front of *Glee*.

Finally, at the end of the day, give yourself a grade on a scale of 1 to 5. If you mark a "1," you've had a bad day, with unhealthy foods. If you write a "5," it was healthy—whatever your current definition of "healthy" is. This scoring can be a reality check: "I'm not doing so badly after all" or "Geez, gotta get in gear here. My diet is worse than I thought."

Logging can be a colossal chore. But it's only for a week, at least to start. Some people struggle to remember to fill it in, especially those who eat frequently. Leslie's clients often leave themselves e-mails or voice mails after they've eaten, and then fill in the form at the end of the day. Find a system that works for you. Just eat as you normally would during these 7 days.

WHY BOTHER?

What's the point of going to the trouble of logging your food? First, even the act of telling yourself "I'm going to write it down" shows a level of commitment to losing weight. If you're purposeful about the log, it means you're serious.

Second, if you don't write it down, you can't begin to get a full picture of your habits and problem areas. Leslie hears her clients say all the time, "I don't understand why I'm not losing weight." They want to point the finger. The fault lies with someone else's cooking or their metabolism slowing when they turned 40 or coworkers who insist on celebrating every birthday. The log shows you who the boss is: You are. When you log, it means you're ready to take a good, hard look at what you're consuming. You're ready to own up.

A food log like this reveals a lot more than what you're eating. If you do it honestly for a week, you'll get an accurate picture of how you eat—quickly or leisurely. It will show you how often you're sitting down with your family or scarfing down dinner in the car on the way home from the school board meeting. It will tell you how many times during the day you eat and how much in each sitting, which might provide clues to why you're hungry again only 2 hours later. Maybe your weekends look completely different from your Monday through Friday. Or if you're eating when you're not hungry, you can ask yourself, *Why is it, exactly, that I'm eating right now?*

You're going to glean some really important information from your log. This makes eating less of an automatic, hand-to-mouth-to-hand-to-mouth activity. Learning about how you eat makes you more mindful. Feeding yourself becomes a purposeful endeavor. Thinking about it will help you see your habits, good and bad.

> The log shows you who the boss is: You are.

Often when people want to lose weight, they change only the food, the "what" they're eating. They'll cut carbs or eat only grapefruit or tuna fish until they can't look at another tuna sandwich as long as they live. In fact, the "what" might not be the problem that's causing them to pack on the pounds. It could be the "when," the "where," the "why," or the "how much." The eating pattern might be what needs to change. But you won't know that until you write it down.

FOR YOUR EYES ONLY

Convinced? Good. Again, this week of logging is meant to give you a snapshot of where you are right now. So don't try to be "extra good" just because you're logging. You're the only one who has to see this.

> Learning about how you eat makes you more mindful.
> Feeding yourself becomes a purposeful endeavor.

In later chapters, we'll address a perfect day of eating—what a "5" day should look like and how to get there. But we're not attacking it all at once.

So how long should you log? Well, at least a week. Studies have shown that people who log their food intake regularly do better with keeping the weight off than those who don't. That's because they're being accountable, and when they're logging, they're thinking about what they're eating.

Most people would find it tedious to log their food every day. Some do it a couple of days a week. Some people record and then stop logging, only to find that logging even for a day or two helps jump-start their weight loss again.

Leslie's Lessons: "Right off the bat, you might be able to see a problem area where you can start changing your eating. It's like tackling a home improvement project. You don't start with the entire house—and you don't start with the entire day. Everyone has a trouble time. For a lot of people, it's nighttime. For others, it's midafternoon. Whatever yours is, that is the one you start to focus on. Don't try to fix the whole day all at once, because that becomes overwhelming."

Food Intake Voyeurism!

Let's see what Leslie eats in a typical day:

TIME	FOOD	AMOUNT	HUNGER
5:30 a.m.	Pear	1 medium	H
	Water	20 oz	
6:30 a.m.	Greek yogurt, vanilla flavored	6 oz	H
	Bran Buds	¼ cup	
	Almonds	2 Tbsp	
	Water	10 oz	
8:30 a.m.	Coffee, black	12 oz	NH
10:00 a.m.	Almonds/raisins	⅓ cup	H
	Green tea	12 oz	
1:00 p.m.	Hummus	⅓ cup	H
	Feta	¼ cup	
	Whole wheat pita	regular size	
	Tomato	2 slices	
	Pickle	1 spear	
	Apple	1 medium	
	Sparkling water	20 oz	
4:00 p.m.	Cheddar cheese	2 oz	H
	Pretzel nuggets	10	
	Sparkling water	20 oz	
8:00 p.m.	Salmon, grilled	5 oz	H
	Salad of mixed greens, peppers, cucumbers, olives, mushrooms	3 cups	
	Fruit (apple, melon, or berries)	¼ cup	
	Olive oil	1 Tbsp	
	Balsamic vinegar	2 Tbsp	
	Red or white wine	5 oz	
	Sparkling water	12 oz	
11:00 p.m.	Water with vitamins	12 oz	NH

MORE HOMEWORK!

There will be less to do in the coming weeks, but first, a few more items to record. You should plan on weighing yourself every week and writing down the number. And there is a proper way to weigh. Try to weigh yourself on the same day of the week at the same time, ideally in the morning. Wake up, use the bathroom, take off your clothes, and step on the scale.

Enter the number here: _____

Enter the number again in the Personal Workbook Week 2 on page 214.

Take some measurements, too. Often when people get into shape, the scale doesn't do them justice. You can actually lose inches off your waist, hips, and thighs, but the pounds don't go down as fast as you'd like. That's because muscle also weighs more than fat. Measurements give you another way to track progress.

So take a tape measure and measure your waist at the thinnest part. Pull the tape measure so it's snug against your body. Guys can usually stop at the waist. Women, you might benefit from doing the same with your chest, hips, and thighs at the widest parts.

Enter the measurements below. We think you'll be pleased when you measure again in 12 weeks.

Waist: _____ inches

Chest: _____ inches

Hips: _____ inches

Thighs: _____ inches

You can enter these numbers in the workbook at the end, too. Now here's that calorie-burning chart I promised you.

CALORIES BURNED PER MILE WALKING OR RUNNING

IF YOU WEIGH:	AND YOU WALK...			AND YOU RUN (THE ENTIRE WAY)...		
	1 MILE	2 MILES	3 MILES	1 MILE	2 MILES	3 MILES
120	63.6	127.2	190.8	90	180	270
130	68.9	137.8	206.7	97.5	195	292.5
140	74.2	148.4	222.6	105	210	315
150	79.5	159	238.5	112.5	225	337.5
160	84.8	169.6	254.4	120	240	360
170	90.1	180.2	270.3	127.5	255	382.5
180	95.4	190.8	286.2	135	270	405
190	100.7	201.4	302.1	142.5	285	427.5
200	106	212	318	150	300	450
210	111.3	222.6	333.9	157.5	315	472.5
220	116.6	233.2	349.8	165	330	495
230	121.9	243.8	365.7	173.5	345	517.5
240	127.2	254.4	381.6	180	360	540
250	132.5	265	397.5	187.5	375	562.5
260	137.8	275.6	413.4	195	390	585
270	143.1	286.2	429.3	202.5	405	607.5
280	148.4	296.8	445.2	210	420	630
290	153.7	307.4	461.1	217.5	435	652.5
300	159	318	477	225	450	675

Calculations based on Cameron, et al., "Energy Expenditure of Walking and Running." *Medicine and Science in Sport and Exercise,* December 2004.

BECKY, 52

Job: Coding claims for an insurance company; mother of two grown children

Goals: Improve my health, lose weight, and achieve a sense of self-accomplishment

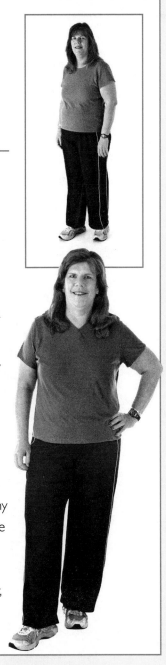

Starting weight: 225 pounds

Ending weight: 212 pounds

Starting waist: 45.5 inches

Ending waist: 41 inches

Words to Live By: "I take nothing for granted. I now only have good days or great days." That's from Lance Armstrong, who is a cancer survivor like me.

Fighting Weak Moments: To aid with my weight loss, I put notes on the fridge and cabinets saying, "Do you want to carry all that weight around with you?" and "You want to carry all that weight up that hill?" That makes me think twice before munching!

Athlete in the Making: I had never done any organized sports of any kind, and now I've done 14 races. I feel great when I run. I feel so fortunate my body is able to do this. I'd like to build up to a 5-miler and a 10-K and, ultimately, a half-marathon.

Chapter 3

Timing Is Everything

As you've seen by now, this running plan is all about gradual. It takes you from walking for 30 minutes to running for 30 minutes in 12 stages.

But just because there are 12 stages doesn't mean you have to do it in 12 weeks. You set the pace. You increase when you're ready. You can stretch this program out over the course of 6 months if that suits you better.

Jeff, who's 42, started the *RYBO* program at 341 pounds. That was a lot of extra weight on a guy who is 5 feet 10 inches. He has always struggled with his weight, but for this busy father of three kids—ages 10, 7, and 5— taking care of himself took a backseat to his job (he is an owner of a stainless steel distributor) and driving to soccer, T-ball, and youth theater. His lower back was killing him, making it hard to do any exercise. The wake-up call came when his family got a Wii and he couldn't stand on the board accessory because the weight limit was 330.

You set the pace.

Jeff started walking: three times the first week, three the next, then he got up to four. Lo and behold, his back pain eased a little. The fourth week, he added a minute of running after every 4 minutes of walking. And he stayed there for 2 weeks. Then he moved up to 2 minutes of running, which, as you'll see on page 42, is this week's workout.

THE SPEED DOESN'T MATTER

Jeff has since progressed to 8 minutes of running and 2 minutes of walking. And he'll be the first to admit that when he runs, he's not threatening any land-speed records. Which is exactly the point: He developed at his own pace. He made his own schedule, often dependent on the heat and humidity of the Pennsylvania summer. He wasn't stuck on increasing his running every week. And some weeks he mixed it up: Monday, Wednesday, and Friday he would do the same workout, and on Saturday he would make it a little easier again: less running, more walking. He also worked with Leslie, going over his food log to see where he could make small changes that would lead to big weight loss.

> Get in the habit of exercising 4 days a week for the rest of your life. There is no stopping at the end of this program.

In 12 weeks, he had dropped 26 pounds.

At the start, his stated goal was to be able to run a mile. Jeff knows it might take him several months to hit that milestone. He's in no rush, nor should he be. He's healthier than he has been in years. He has a long way to go to get to his ideal weight, but he's well on his way.

So there's a fine line. Yes, you want to push yourself a little bit. You want to run more. If you get stuck in a walking rut, you won't get the benefit of the additional calorie-burning that we discussed in the last chapter.

At the same time, you don't want to push so hard that you find yourself discouraged and quit. That would be terrible! We're hoping you'll get in the habit of exercising 4 days a week for the rest of your life. There is no stopping at the end of this program.

It's common with new runners and exercisers that something happens to subvert their week, and they fall off the wagon. Maybe it's the flu, maybe it's a work deadline, maybe it's an unexpected trip out of state to look in on your elderly aunt. You don't get your three or four workouts in.

The mistake is to try to climb back on the wagon at the exact same place where you fell off or, worse, to try to increase the intensity without having done your homework. Make sure you've laid the groundwork before you try to build up the running interval. When you're ready, take it up a notch.

Here we go with the third stage.

Budd's Buzz: "The point is the consistency. Don't step it up until you get a solid week in at one level. I usually tell people to step back a week from their last training session if they've been sick. If they moved from 1 minute of running and 4 of walking to 2 minutes of running and 4 of walking, they should go back to 1 minute of running. If that's too easy after their first session back, they can resume running 2, walking 4."

STAGE 3 WORKOUT

- Walk for 4 minutes. Run for 2 minutes.

- Repeat that sequence four more times.

- End with 3 minutes of walking.

Total workout time: 33 minutes, 10 of which are running.

Do this workout at least three or four times in a week before
moving on to the next stage.

The same rules apply from the previous chapter:

- Go very slowly.

- Try not to be huffing and puffing. If you are, you're going too fast.

- Think of running as no faster than your walk.

Got it? Good.

Meanwhile, in the personal workbook at the end of this book, you'll see
an exercise log. This is actually a fun document. And we've included additional exercise log pages for you to use when you've completed the workbook. You can enter the date, the workout you did, and the total time you
were out there and what portion of it was running. You'll notice spaces for
a few comments. Write about the weather, if the day felt easier or harder
than you expected, if you spotted any wildlife, or if last night's fish was
coming back to haunt you.

Do you have to keep a log? No. But you might enjoy it. If you keep filling
it in, in a few weeks or months you can take a look back and see how much
progress you've made in a relatively short time. It can be exciting to see those
pages fill up with workouts, especially if you were sedentary before.

And when you're mixing and matching workouts, say, three Stage 3
workouts and one Stage 1 workout this week, you can keep track of what
you've done in the exercise log. I know I find it hard to remember what I

did this morning, let alone last Monday. Put your weight in at the end of each week, and you'll have a good record of all you've accomplished.

Also, you can use the log to enter any other extra activity beyond your baseline. Have a regular squash game with Bert from accounting? Put that in. If you do yoga or toning exercises, enter them. If you like to swim laps, put that in there. If you took the dogs on a 5-mile hike, in that goes.

I love my logs. I've got them stacked up in a closet going back years, but I rarely look at them. I think it's the entering and then tallying of the miles at the end of the week that gives me a moment of satisfaction. On the good weeks, it gives me a boost to look back and see that there's only one empty space. On the bad weeks, when the kids are sick or the babysitter cancels or work is nuts, I write that in there, too, usually with a sad face emoticon. (These aren't deep thoughts I'm recording.) But even if the dirty laundry is overflowing the basket, the editors are clamoring for a story, and the dust on the TV screen makes the picture fuzzy, well, I've got my log. It's my own way of saying "At least I got something done today."

So the 7 days of food logging? That's mandatory. The exercise log? That's pure fun. Enjoy it.

 ## Extra Credit

If you're used to doing other activity, keep it up! The more active you are, the more calories you burn. Don't think that just because you're starting to run, you have to quit all your other activities. Runners just call other sports cross-training, and they're good for you. They work muscle groups that you might not hit with running and give you a mental break in your routine when you have something different to anticipate. Plus, you might notice that walking and running are already helping those endeavors. Maybe you're not exhausted anymore after a long set of tennis.

You'll notice that each stage of the beginning running program begins with a walk. This is a warmup, and it prepares your muscles, heart, and lungs for the more demanding periods of running that are part of each workout.

Some beginning runners like to stretch even before they walk. Do you have to stretch? It's up to you. It's important to remember, however, not to stretch cold muscles, because you risk injuring yourself. It's best to get moving with an active warmup, like this "dynamic flexibility" series below. Save your "static" stretching for when you're finished with your workout and your muscles are warm. Here are Budd's suggestions for warmup and cooldown routines. Remember to keep it gentle during the warmup!

WARMUP: DYNAMIC FLEXIBILITY

1. **Hip circle:** Stand with your feet shoulder-width apart. Circle your hips as if you were attempting to hula-hoop. Perform eight rotations in one direction, then eight in the opposite direction.

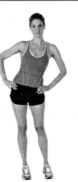
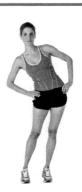

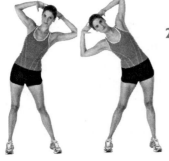

2. **Body lean:** With your feet slightly more than shoulder-width apart and your fingers touching behind your head, lean side to side from left to right. Start with very gentle leans. Do eight repetitions and go a little deeper after the first few.

3. Forward leg swing: Place your right hand on a stationary object, like a wall or a pole, for balance. With your knee almost straight and your foot flexed gently, swing your left leg forward and backward. Repeat with the right leg, doing eight repetitions on each side.

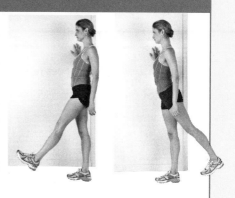

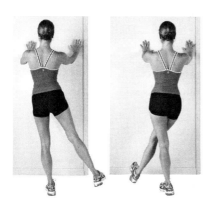

4. Lateral leg swing: Stand facing a wall about 18 inches away. Place your hands on the wall at shoulder height. With your right knee straight and your right foot flexed, swing your right leg out to the side, then back in front of your left leg. Do eight repetitions, then repeat with the left leg.

5. Heel raises: Stand with your feet shoulder-width apart. Gently rise up onto your tiptoes, then slowly come back down. Rock back onto your heels and let your toes come off the ground. Repeat eight times.

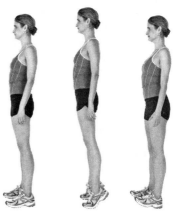

(continued on page 46)

COOLDOWN

1. **Lower back and hamstring stretch:** Stand with your feet shoulder-width apart and your hands clasped behind your back. Keep your legs straight and bend over as far as you can while raising your clasped hands behind you as high as you can. Hold this position for a count of 8. While in this position, gently release your 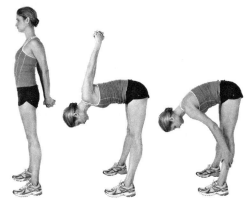 hands and reach down and grasp behind your lower legs. Pull slightly to extend the stretch and hold for another 8 seconds. Bend your knees, release your hands, and stand up.

2. **Basic calf stretch:** Stand with your feet shoulder-width apart and a little more than arm's length from a stationary object such as a wall, tree, or pole. Reach your arms forward at shoulder height and lean so you're touching the wall. Bring your left foot forward so your left toes are nearly touching the wall, then bend your left knee. Keep your right foot flat on the ground and your right knee straight. This stretches your right calf. If you don't feel the stretch in your right calf, try moving your hips toward the wall and bending your arms. Hold this stretch for 8 seconds and repeat on the opposite side.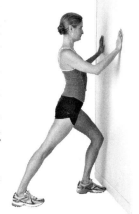

3. Calf stretch variation: Repeat the basic calf stretch, but this time bend your rear leg slightly. This moves the stretch down your leg and closer to your foot.

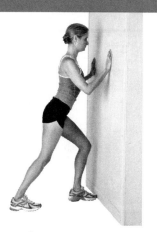

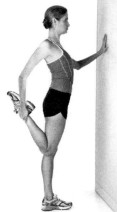

4. Quad stretch: Stand with your feet shoulder-width apart near a stationary object, like a wall or a pole, for balance. Support yourself against the wall with your left arm. Reach back with your right hand and grasp your right ankle behind you so you bring your heel up near your rear end. Raise your knee behind you as far as possible. Hold for 8 seconds, then repeat on the opposite side.

5. Hip and iliotibial band stretch: Stand with your feet together and your right side facing a wall or pole slightly more than arm's length away. Extend your arm out straight and lean so your palm is on the wall. Keeping your legs and arm straight, push your hips toward the wall. Hold that position for about 8 seconds. Repeat on the opposite side.

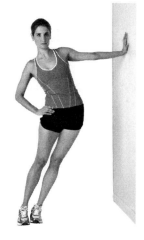

FOOD TALK Space It!

As Leslie told us in the previous chapter, you get to wheel and deal with your eating several times a day. If you can learn to evenly space out the time you're eating, you'll reach the point of desperate hunger less frequently, and you can easily shed a couple of hundred calories. We doubt you'll even notice they're gone.

Get out your log and take a look at the "when." Are you eating at regular intervals throughout the day? Or do you nibble until you're home from work and then down everything you can get your hands on?

BAD TIMING

This, according to Leslie, is a classic case of "uploading": We're so busy during the day that we don't eat enough. When we finally do have time to eat at night, it's off to the races, finishing dinner, then scavenging in the cupboards, fridge, and freezer.

In an ideal world you'd have three meals, each about the same size. Breakfast is maybe a little smaller, dinner maybe a little more. Then you get a decent-size snack, either in the afternoon if you're eating late or in the evening if you've eaten dinner early. A second small snack, if necessary, can tide you over between breakfast and lunch.

But when you only eat little nibbles throughout the day, you're exhausted from hunger. And then you're setting yourself up to overdo it with a giant meal at night.

HOW THE TIMING LOOKS ON A GOOD DAY

Here are two possible timing scenarios for a sensible day of eating. Obviously, you can adjust them to fit your schedule, but you can see how the meals occur at regular intervals throughout the day.

7:00 a.m.: Breakfast

10:00 a.m.: Small snack, if necessary

12 noon or 1:00 p.m.: Lunch, depending on whether you had a morning snack

4:00 p.m.: Snack

8:00 p.m.: Dinner

SCENARIO 2

7:00 a.m.: Breakfast

10:00 a.m.: Small snack, if necessary

12 noon or 1:00 p.m.: Lunch, depending on whether you had a morning snack

5:30 p.m.: Dinner

9:30 p.m.: Snack

BREAKFAST ADVISORY

Look, if you're realistically going to be able to make it for 4 to 5 hours without eating after breakfast, you have to eat a decent-size meal. Otherwise you'll be sitting in your 10:00 a.m. meeting feeling like you're going to pass out.

Try to eat breakfast within 1 hour of waking up. If you work out in the morning, split breakfast. Have a little something before you go, like half a banana, and finish eating when you've finished your run.

Eating breakfast is crucial for three reasons. First, it "breaks" the overnight "fast" and gets the body started in the process of digesting again. Second, it's damage control. Eat breakfast and you won't be so hungry later on that you go overboard with your other meals. Third, breakfast provides your body with nutrients you need, both for exercise and just to function throughout the day. According to the National Weight Control Registry of people who have lost 30 pounds and successfully kept it off for a year or longer, 88 percent of them eat breakfast at least 5 days a week.

RANT ALERT!

One test panelist who dropped out before completing the study told me how she had to get up by 6:00 a.m. every day, get her 4-year-old son off to daycare, and then work full-time. She usually skipped breakfast at home, maybe nibbling on a few almonds on the way to work. She had a granola bar around 11:00 a.m. Lunch was some mixed raw vegetables dipped in hummus. It sounds healthy, but it was next to nothing. At night, when she finally had time to relax, she'd overdo it with a large dinner. And she wondered why the weight wasn't coming off.

When Leslie talked to her about breakfast, she wasn't ready to hear it. "I'm just going to cut out carbs for a while," she told me.

Eating breakfast is crucial.

Excuse me while I vent. That sort of thinking—or, rather, lack of thinking—is really frustrating. Entirely eliminating a category of foods, such as carbs, is not sustainable in the long haul. It might give you a quick start to your weight loss, but it won't last. It's only changing the "what," not the "when" or "where."

The lessons here are meant to train your brain as well as your mouth. If you're going to lose weight and keep it off, you have to think, not just eat.

Okay, rant over.

> Entirely eliminating a category of foods, such as carbs, is not sustainable in the long haul. It might give you a quick start to your weight loss, but it won't last very long.

BACK TO BREAKFAST

Here are three ways to get a substantial, well-balanced breakfast without dirtying a whole bunch of dishes:

1. Have a bowl of high-fiber cereal with ½ cup of fat-free milk and a serving of cottage cheese on the side.

2. Make oatmeal in the microwave, using milk instead of water. Top with 2 tablespoons of nuts and half an apple, sliced.

3. Toast a whole wheat English muffin. Put a slice of low-fat cheese on one side and a slice of ham on the other to make a breakfast sandwich.

While we're at it, check out five Leslie-approved breakfast cereals:

- Oatmeal

- Kellogg's Raisin Bran

- Kellogg's All-Bran Bran Buds

- General Mills Fiber One

- Kashi Cinnamon Harvest

Experiment with eating a little more at breakfast this week. See what you notice. You might be surprised by how long you go before you start feeling hunger pangs.

STEPHANIE, 39

Job: Stay-at-home mom of two kids.

Goals: To lose weight and be able to play with my kids in a more active way

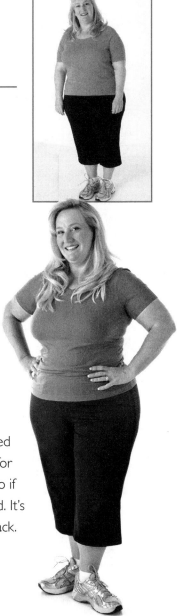

Starting weight: 231 pounds

Ending weight: 219 pounds

Starting waist: 38 inches

Ending waist: 35 inches

When Facing Temptation: I try to think about how good it feels to fit in smaller clothes and look good in them. When I don't feel like working out, I remind myself how great it feels once I'm done.

Breakfast Struggle: It's a challenge for me to eat breakfast, because I'm just not hungry in the morning. I wake up by 6:30 or 7:00, but I'm not usually hungry until 9:00 or 10:00. So now I force myself to have at least a banana.

Guilt-Free Nighttime Snacking: I've learned it's okay to have a snack at night. I'm usually up for another 2 or 3 hours after my kids go to bed. So if we had dinner at 5:30, I'll be starving before bed. It's great not to feel guilty about a small evening snack.

My First Race: It was very satisfying! I went with Dorene the Friday before to check out the course and make sure we could do it, and when we finished it, we looked at each other like, "Really? We just did it." Then on race day, we basically ran the whole thing. There were a few times when we power-walked, but Dorene would let us do only about 30 seconds before she had us running again. When we finished, with all those cheering people, it was very uplifting. They really make you feel like it's a major accomplishment.

Power Tool: My slow cooker is my best friend. My kids get home from school at 4:00 p.m., then one has swimming from 5:00 to 6:00 p.m., and the other swims from 6:00 to 7:30. We're in and out. I would love to sit down and have dinner together, but it doesn't always happen for us. With the slow cooker, I can make something healthy in the morning, and it's ready when we want it. I make a lot of soups because I can control the vegetables and spices and make sure that there's not a whole lot of extra sodium.

Inspiring the Family: My kids and my husband watched me go through the process of training for a race, and they learned it was a lot of hard work and it doesn't just happen. I think my kids internalized that lesson. If they want to achieve a sports goal or a school goal, they have to put in the effort in their 8-year-old and 10-year-old ways. I'm proud of showing them that.

THE NEW RULE ON EATING AT NIGHT

Notice how in the second meal-timing scenario, you're allowed a late-night snack. This differs from many weight-loss plans, which strictly forbid eating after 7:00 p.m. Yes, you read that right. It's not a typo. Depending on your schedule, a light meal a few hours after dinner can be fine.

Blasphemy, you say? Well, what if you eat with your kids at 5:30 and stay up until 11:00? You'll be starved before you go to bed. Suppose you exercise at night? You'll need a little something after your workout. And many folks find they sleep better if they eat a snack at night.

The key here is to think about what you're doing at night. Really put some thought into it. Are you hungry because it has been several hours since dinner, or is it that you're just used to munching while you watch TV? If it's the former, go for a good snack. If it's the latter, put away the chips and ice cream, go brush your teeth, and do something else until you're ready for bed.

Think about what you're doing at night.

What makes a good after-dinner snack? Look closely at Leslie's suggestions here and you'll notice they are an awful lot like breakfast. They include fiber and protein, and they require the use of silverware, which means they're premeditated snacks. There's no reaching into a bag for a handful of this or that as you coast through the kitchen on the way to the laundry room.

SENSIBLE EVENING SNACKS

- Mix ¼ cup of Bran Buds cereal in a serving of yogurt.

- Toast a whole grain waffle and top it with 1 tablespoon of preserves or maple syrup. Have it with a 6-ounce glass of fat-free milk.

- Slice an apple and eat it with 1 tablespoon of peanut butter.

FORGET ABOUT GRAZING

A few years back, "grazing" came into vogue in dieting circles. The idea was that instead of eating three meals a day, you'd eat six small meals. The rationale seemed okay: You'd never let yourself get too hungry, and then you wouldn't overdo at any one meal.

But in reality, grazing doesn't work. We're Americans, and we have trouble doing anything small. So this plan quickly backfired. Six small meals turned into six large ones. We were eating constantly throughout

Leslie's Lessons: "Grazing doesn't work for so many reasons. It isn't necessarily multinutrient—usually it's just crackers or cookies or fruit, because most people don't graze on vegetables or chicken. If one constantly grazes on carbs, more bacteria are produced in the mouth, which can cause tooth decay. And with grazing, the body never knows when to stop. How can you know if you are hungry or full when you're constantly exposed to food? The mind goes out of the equation, and you're just exercising your mouth. Without a pause in eating, you're always starting the digestive cascade, with the increased salivary secretion and digestive enzymes constantly stimulating the gut. The appetite switch is always on. It's not a pretty picture."

the day—a bite here, a handful there. And we packed on the pounds even faster. Cattle graze; people shouldn't.

Changing the timing of what you eat can be tough to get used to at first. If you're not accustomed to a big breakfast, it can take several days to build up to it. When you're constantly snacking throughout the day and you instead try to aggregate your eating occasions around three meals and a snack, you might find yourself experiencing hunger pangs at those times when you used to grab a handful of pretzels.

The goal is to eat when you're hungry but not starving, so you don't overdo it in one sitting. No doubt the timing and the quantities will be a work in progress for a couple of weeks. But you'll likely find that you consume fewer total calories throughout the day. And that's what you need to do to shed weight. Remember, the calories you burn must exceed the calories you take in each day.

> The goal is to eat when you're hungry but not starving.

HOW TO SET GOALS

Before our test panel participants began this study, we asked them to fill out a questionnaire, which included lines for three goals. Even though the folks were of all different ages and sizes and occupations, their goals were strikingly similar. As I flipped through the paperwork, I saw the same goals pop up over and over.

1. Lose weight.

2. Feel better.

A few of the participants added a running goal. They wanted to be able to jog a local 5-K or run a mile without stopping.

Those are all perfectly fine goals. But we think they could be more focused.

We like goals that have a time frame and a number on them.

We like goals that have a time frame and a number on them. That way, they're measurable. You can check back in on yourself at the end of the allotted time and say either "Yes, I've accomplished that goal" or "No, I'm halfway to my goal and I'll give myself another month."

Let's look at how we could revise the goals above to have measurable results and a deadline. The "lose weight" goal is easy. Knowing what we know now—namely, that ½ to 1 pound per week of weight loss is what the experts recommend—you could say to yourself that you want to lose 8 pounds in 3 months. You know what your weight is now; subtract 8, look at the calendar, and circle that date.

But "feel better"? That's a toughie. What exactly do you mean by that? We think we have an idea. You want to sleep more soundly at night, you want to hit 2:00 p.m. and not feel like you need a nap, you want to keep up with your kids. So how's this: Instead of simply writing "feel better," think of a surefire way you'll *know* when you feel better. You'll be able to hike up the mountain near where your family vacations every August. You'll be able to walk the mall for your holiday shopping and get it all done in a day. You'll be able to climb the jungle gym with your 2-year-old before July 4. You want to be able to kick the blood pressure medication in 6 months. (That's a great goal and a true measure of better health, but you need to do it under your doctor's supervision.)

In fact, Jeff initially set his goal as running a mile, but he realized midway through the program that he had another goal. He vacations with his

---

Leslie's Lessons: "If you're in Week 1, then Week 52 looks awfully far away. Set a goal in a shorter time frame. Then get engaged in the process. All of us tend to respond better when we have a carrot dangling in front of us."

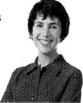

family at Disney World every year. "In the past I have struggled with all the walking that's required," he says. "This year I want to keep up."

Wow. That's a cool one.

The point is this: Give yourself specific goals and a target date for meeting them. Then you can see how you've done and know if it's time to set new ones.

Why has it taken us until the end of the third chapter to talk about goals? Well, we figure before you can set the right goals, you need a little knowledge. You need some objective data about where you are now before you can decide where you want to be in the future. Now you know your weight and activity level. You know what a reasonable rate of weight loss is.

So here are four lines. You don't have to fill them all, but put in at least one goal that has to do with your weight and one that has to do with your running. You can also enter them in Personal Workbook Week 3. Have at it.

_____

_____

_____

_____

Now that you've set your goals, the next step is establishing a plan for getting there. We think the knowledge Budd and Leslie share in the upcoming chapters will help you develop your plan. At the end

---

Budd's Buzz: "Publicize your goals. Tell your spouse, your kids, your friends, and they'll ask, 'How ya doing on that?' And you have to report back to them. You're asking them to participate in your weight loss and your running, so they won't be so likely to nudge the cake in your direction or infringe on your workout time."

of the book, you can write down your plan for meeting your goals.

A quick example to get your gears turning: Let's say you want to lose 2 pounds this month. That's a 7,000-calorie deficit, which works out to a 225-calorie deficit per day if there are 31 days in the month. So how exactly are you going to create that deficit? Cut from 2 percent milk to fat-free, skip the dessert, walk and run 3 miles on 4 days each week? You can see how your goals can lead to a well-designed plan.

In the meantime, make a copy of your goals and put them somewhere you'll see them frequently—your bathroom mirror, your desk, the fridge.

Okay, then, the three of us will do it, too. Boy, this is getting personal!

Leslie's Goals

Do some form of exercise 7 days a week.

Cook something in the kitchen at least once a day.

Actively challenge my brain in a new way at least once a day.

Budd's Goals

Win my age group at the Pittsburgh Marathon.

Keep my body fat to 7 percent or less.

Eat evenly throughout the day so I'm not snacking too much late at night.

Sarah's Goals

Break 43 minutes at the New York Mini 10-K in June.

Weigh 130 pounds on New Year's Day.

Snack less between meals so I have no more cavities.

DORENE, 47

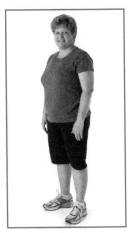

Job: Stay-at-home mom of a 10-year-old; active volunteer

Goals: To lose weight and learn to enjoy running so I'll be motivated to continue even after the program is over

Starting weight: 193 pounds

Ending weight: 174 pounds

Starting waist: 41 inches

Ending waist: 37 inches

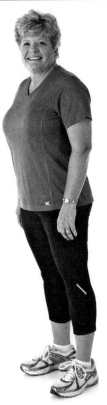

Going through My Head: No music—usually if I'm running with Stephanie, we talk. If I'm alone, I spend the time as personal time—thinking, praying, and checking out all the sights around me.

New Goals: I would like to lose another 20 pounds. And I want to break 35 minutes for a 5-K. I've always loved sports, so it's easy for me to get in the mind-set of competing with myself. I played field hockey and lacrosse, and I was a physical education teacher before I had my son. It used to be that if I was on a field, I could run until I dropped. But put me on a track, and I hated it. That's changed. I enjoy running now, and I miss it if I can't get out there.

When I'm Confronted by Unhealthy Food: I think to myself, *God, give me strength!* Then I think about the weight I would like the scale to read the next day.

What Worked the Most: Spacing my meals. I used to snack with my son when he got home from school, so it was a big change not to eat then. If I am really hungry at that time, I make sure it's a healthy snack like a Kashi granola bar.

Start Slow: When Stephanie and I first started running, we were going too fast. I'd advise beginning runners not to get caught up in anyone else's pace. Tune in to what your body is saying. Slow should be your slow, not anyone else's idea of slow.

Chapter 4

"Running is a big question mark that's there each and every day. It asks you, 'Are you going to be a wimp, or are you going to be strong today?'" —Peter Maher, two-time Olympic marathoner from Canada

Sticking with It

Julie started on the test panel in April 2010, carrying 181 pounds on her 5-foot-4 frame. She's like a lot of 38-year-old women: busy with a career, two kids, and a husband. Pretty much the last thing she thinks about is herself.

She had made various halfhearted (and some full-hearted) attempts at losing weight in the past. She's a lifetime member of Weight Watchers but had stopped going regularly; instead, she was walking at the local high school track 3 evenings a week.

> After a few weeks she started to look forward to running. "It grew on me," she says. "It became my *me* time."

Then some of her colleagues at work mentioned they were signing up for First Strides, a popular beginning running program here in Pennsylvania's Lehigh Valley. Julie couldn't make the course fit into her schedule, but her coworkers came back excited about it, and something clicked in her brain. She needed a goal, a way to focus her weight-loss efforts. She had often thought about participating in a 3-day, 60-mile breast cancer walk that takes place in Philadelphia but figured, "There's no way I could do that." But when she heard about our study, she decided it was manageable enough, at least to start.

She ran at night because it was the only time she could fit it in. At first her breathing felt too hard, and she struggled to get through the running segments. After talking with Budd, who told her to slow down, she began to get the hang of it. Her daughters, who came along with her and sat in the bleachers while she ran, were very encouraging. "Mom, we can't believe you're doing this. You look great," they told her. Her husband was impressed—flabbergasted is more like it. After a few weeks, she started to look forward to running. "It grew on me," she says. "It became my *me* time."

In her 10th week of running, Julie realized she could run 13 minutes without stopping. That night she signed up for her first race. She had been meaning to do it later in the fall. But with her newfound enthusiasm and

13 pounds thinner, she figured, why wait? "I never would have guessed I would do this," she says. "Who, at 38 years old, decides they're going to start running? And I did!"

HOW SLOW CAN YOU GO?

If you're doing these workouts correctly, there is not a big shift in speed from the walk to the run. You're running at about the pace of a brisk walk. And you shouldn't be getting too out of breath. If you are, slow it down. "That was my biggest problem at first," Julie says. "I got winded so easily, and that's really discouraging. I think what made it stick for me was forgetting about speed and focusing on keeping my breathing under control. Once I was able to do that, it was easier to add more time to each running segment."

> If you sense that people are taking a long look at you as you run by, it's probably because they admire your effort. You're out there doing something for yourself. They wish they had the courage to run.

YEAH, BUT THAT'S EMBARRASSING!

Some people start to jog and get all embarrassed by their slow pace. And their jiggling. But really, you shouldn't be shy. People who you think are passing judgment usually aren't. If you sense that people are taking a long look at you as you run by, it's probably because they admire your effort. You're out there doing something for yourself. They wish they had the courage to run.

A lot of new runners think that running is an exclusive club, and they don't belong if they can't achieve a certain speed. That's nonsense, and it's self-defeating. Don't worry about anyone else. Worry about *you*. You're the one taking control of your health, which puts you in a select group. With much of America overweight, pretty soon you'll be the authority, the one people are coming to for tips. Plus, if you can stick it out for 12 weeks or so, you'll get faster without even realizing it. It's simply a natural development as you grow more fit.

Still embarrassed? Take a hint from our test panelist Becky, who survived stage III colon cancer. Think she gives a damn what people say about her running? "Hey, I'm out here," she says. "I'm trying. And you know what? I'm happy doing it."

STAGE 4 WORKOUT

- Walk for 3 minutes. Run for 3 minutes.

- Repeat that sequence four more times.

- End with 3 minutes of walking.

Total workout time: 33 minutes, 15 of which are running.

Do this workout at least three or four times in a
week before moving on to the next stage.

You're halfway there! If you can run for 15 minutes at a time, that's a big deal. And if you do this workout four times a week, you'll be running an hour this week. That probably didn't seem too likely a few weeks back, did it?

STRESS, RELAX, STRESS AGAIN: A LITTLE BACKGROUND ON THIS PLAN

You might not have realized this, but your training is guided by the same principle Olympians use for their training. You have something in common with the great American women's marathon record holder Deena Kastor and Michael Phelps, owner of 14 Olympic swimming medals.

Each time you run, you put your body through a period of stress. That stress interval is followed by a recovery phase, which is the walking portion. Then you repeat that pattern: stress, recover, stress, recover. This is the same pattern at work in the programs elite athletes follow, whether they're runners, cyclists, or swimmers. They have hard days and they have easy days in their training. And on their hard days, they do interval training: periods of stress followed by a recovery time, then stress again. For an elite runner, the workout might be five 1-mile repeats with 400-meter jogs in between. But it's the same idea that you're applying here. (Just wanted to give you a little confidence in case you were worried that Budd was pulling this out of thin air.)

> Each time you run, you put your body through a period of stress. That stress interval is followed by a recovery phase, which is the walking portion.

Budd knows his stuff. He's been using variants of this plan for 30 years with beginning runners who are employees of Rodale. This plan is the foundation of First Strides, which gets hundreds of women running for the first time every year. Don't doubt Budd.

For us mere mortals, it's important not to get freaked out by the term "stress." As we keep saying, running shouldn't feel that hard. As time goes on, the periods of stress become longer and the recovery portion becomes shorter, until you're able to run nonstop for 30 minutes.

You'll also notice that the running segments feel easier. One minute of running might have been tough at first, but when you're doing 3 minutes, that first minute goes by without a thought. See? You're getting in shape already.

Take a few minutes to write down some thoughts on running so far.

Do you like it? Does it feel awkward? Is it easier than it was a few weeks back? Do you have any hang-ups?

_____

_____

_____

_____

TRICKS OF THE TREADMILL

Ideally, you're getting outside for your runs, breathing in fresh air, noticing birds and flowers, and chatting with your friends. But if you're running indoors on a treadmill, that's okay, too.

Treadmills have a lot going for them. They give you a place to work out when it's 35 degrees outside and the rain is blowing sideways. If you're parked in front of a TV, you have a built-in distraction. They offer a soft, flat surface for running where you don't have to worry about traffic, dogs, kids on bikes, or errant golf balls. All of these are great reasons to use a treadmill, either at home or at a gym, when the conditions outside are less than ideal.

Beginning runners often wonder whether they get the same workout on a treadmill as they do outdoors. It's easier for your foot to push off a

Budd's Buzz: "You don't want to pay a whole lot of attention to how fast you're going on a treadmill. Use your own sense of effort to guide your speed. Put a towel over the console. When you want to speed up, stick your finger on the button under the towel and increase the speed to the point where you feel comfortable running. Don't look at the number. Don't get sucked in at a pace the preset program on the treadmill tells you to go or a pace you think you should be going."

treadmill than it is, say, a dirt path. You don't have to deal with wind resistance. Sometimes it feels easier. To which we say, "Who cares?" At the beginning runner level, it's perfectly fine to substitute a treadmill workout for your regularly scheduled outdoor workout.

Here's the problem, though. Beginners get caught up in the data on the console: the calories burned, the miles covered, the speed. At this stage in your development as a runner, it's not healthy to fixate on the numbers. Say you do the Stage 3 workout and you cover 2.3 miles. But the next time you try it, you only make it 2.2. No biggie! Ignore that!

FRIEND REQUEST

More than any piece of equipment, what's the one thing that's really going to help you stick with this program?

A buddy. One with two legs, not four.

Now, this doesn't mean you'll fail if you can't find anyone to tag along. A number of people—like Harrison, our test panelist who lost 11 pounds—did it all by their lonesome. So did Julie. Budd is usually a solo runner. So is Leslie.

But knowing a friend is out there waiting for you can make all the difference between whether you hit the "snooze" button or get out of bed. That's what we learned from Dorene and Stephanie, who combined to lose 31 pounds. "I probably would not have been as faithful to the program if I hadn't had to be accountable to someone else," Stephanie says. "There was this unspoken feeling of 'Okay, we did this together. If you're not going to do your homework, then you're letting me down.' So we truly were like a team coming through it. And it's so valuable just to have someone you can talk to about what you're struggling with."

I'm normally a solo runner myself, but on weekends I need the nudge of another person to get my lazy butt out of bed. If I'm facing a Saturday morning full of busy activities, I'll call my friend Carla, and we'll coordinate to meet at a trail at 6:30 a.m. Otherwise, the run is just not going to

Budd's Buzz: "When you have a friend going through the program with you, you can discuss your progress. As you do each stage together, you can pat each other on the back. You get more than camaraderie during the run; you get that instant feedback: 'Wow! We did it today!' When you're on your own, you might be the only one who notices. And a buddy is a distraction. You talk to each other rather than overthinking every step, like you might do if you're alone."

happen for me on a Saturday. The thought of Carla doing the same thing, getting out of bed and driving somewhere to meet me, gets me up.

As your running improves and the length of time you can run each week increases, you've got a lot to be proud of. Remember, though, we're still at an early stage, when it's easier to cut more calories by eating correctly than it is to burn more calories with intense runs.

FOOD TALK — Measure It!

Get out the bowl you usually use for breakfast cereal. Fill it as you normally would with the cereal of your choice, say, raisin bran. Now read the label on the box to find out how much is in a serving.

Look at what's in the bowl. Is that more than a 1-cup serving? Less? Do you honestly have any idea? Pull out a measuring cup, dump in the contents of the bowl, and see.

It's a lot more, huh? You're not alone in that. So many of us measure servings with our eyes, and our eyes are terrible judges of portions.

This week, you calculate your calorie intake for a typical day. Eating right requires some detective work and a little forethought. With practice you will be able to eyeball an appropriate serving size. For now, you need the tools.

MEASURE EVERYTHING

Get out all your measuring cups, the ones for dry ingredients and wet. Collapsible measuring cups from Target or Bed Bath & Beyond are a good investment because you can stick them right in the box of cereal or pasta.

As you go through your week, try to read the label on everything you eat and measure out a true serving size. The grains tend to be the hardest: pasta, rice, cereal, and so on. And every brand has a different serving size. Cheerios, for instance, is a cup, but many granola servings are only ½ cup. And if you tried to eat a cup of Grape-Nuts, your jaw would be in

> Eating right requires some detective work and a little forethought.

traction! But it's well worth educating yourself about portions, because those cereals and grains are often the "big-ticket items" that will run up your calorie count very quickly.

Juice is tricky, too. Although a serving of Tropicana orange juice is 8 ounces, other varieties set a serving at 4 or 6 ounces. Look out for snack foods like nuts, crackers, chips, and pretzels. You'll actually have to measure ¼ cup of nuts and start counting your pretzels. Condiments, especially salad dressing, are a sore spot, as are cream cheese and peanut butter. I guarantee, unless we're measuring or eating something that comes prepackaged in a single-serving size, we're all eating more of these than one serving.

Here's what you do:

- Leave the measuring cups out on the counter so you remember to use them all week.

Leslie's Lessons: "No handfuls! My clients are always telling me they had a handful of nuts. Well, how big is your hand? Unless you've got a hand shaped like a measuring cup, there's no way to know."

- Put a collapsible cup in the box of your favorite breakfast cereal.

- Plan to measure out proper portions of condiments. For salad dressing, the serving size is usually 2 tablespoons.

- Make sure you can still see the bread peeking out after you've spread peanut butter or cream cheese. Reduced-fat peanut butter has the same number of calories per serving as regular.

- Try adding water or seltzer to stretch out a serving size of juice that looks puny in your cup.

- Read the label on snack foods. Either count out the crackers or divide the box evenly into serving sizes, and store each serving in an airtight container.

- Read the label on a block of cheese to find out how many servings are in the package, then score the cheese appropriately.

Sure, this will be tedious. It may be annoying. But it's really hard to lose weight if you don't have an accurate idea of your consumption.

TRAIN YOUR BRAIN

Many of the fad diets that have been popular over the past decade have completely eliminated a particular type of food or food group or overloaded on a strange ingredient. First everything was fat-free. Then there was the oat bran craze. Carbs got the boot when Atkins came along. The only thing that all these plans had in common? People didn't have to think. They could just keep shoveling in the calories as long as they were eating or avoiding the one item that each particular diet zeroed in on.

Look, you need to train the muscle between your ears as much as your stomach and legs. You have to think this through if you're going to be able to make the choices that will help you lose weight. *RYBO*, remember, is about education, not deprivation. When you're at the store, you have to learn to do the flip-and-read—the glance at the label—to understand what you're getting.

> Today's bowls, plates, and cups are so enormous that a true serving size is dwarfed.

For instance, the recommended serving size of pasta is usually ½ cup cooked. And that's not very much. If you want to eat two servings or more, fine. But be aware that you're eating two. (An Italian restaurant might plop 6 cups in front of you, which is 12 servings!) Later, after a few weeks of all this measuring, your eyes and brain will learn what a serving size looks like. For now, you'll likely discover that a serving size is far less than what you normally eat.

Adding to the problem? Today's bowls, plates, and cups are so enormous that a true serving size is dwarfed. You have to buy kids' cups to make that serving of juice look like it will be satisfying. I know this is reality. When my husband and I got married and we registered at Crate & Barrel, the "everyday" plates and bowls we chose were huge. The cereal bowls are almost like mixing bowls. Later on, when we were looking to buy our first home, some of the cupboards in older houses weren't deep enough to hold the dinner plates we got as wedding gifts in 2002. Leslie, who got married in 1979, would love to buy new dishes, but she refuses to buy 12-inch dinner plates. "Those aren't plates, they're troughs," she says.

Keep your small plates handy. Eat dinner off a salad plate if you have to. Think a little before you eat.

COUNT THE CALORIES FOR A DAY

If you're still keeping a food log, this is a good time to count the calories you're eating. If you're not, write down everything you eat for 1 day—a typical day—and then go back and figure out how many calories you consumed. CalorieKing.com is a great site for assigning calories to foods because it includes a wide span of brands. Leslie also recommends the food tracker at MyPyramid.gov. Click on the "Analyze My Diet" link.

Here's a place where you can tally your numbers. Personal Workbook Week 4 takes you through this process also.

BREAKFAST:	CALORIES
LUNCH:	
DINNER:	
SNACKS (IF APPLICABLE):	
TOTAL:	

Take a look at that total. Is it above your Harris-Benedict BMR from back in Chapter 1, below your BMR, or right around it? Are your calories divided evenly throughout the day, or are you eating a huge meal at one particular time?

You can see now where you can start to play with the numbers. Remember, to lose 1 pound of fat a week, you need a deficit of about 500 calories per day. If you want to lose ½ pound a week, you need a deficit of 250 per day.

On the days that you're doing an early stage *RYBO* workout, you can figure you're burning somewhere between 150 to 250 extra calories there. The rest has to come from food decisions.

I HATE PUTTING NUMBERS ON FOOD

Calorie counting is a chore, which is why we recommend doing it only once or twice. It gets ridiculous if you start counting calories every day for 3 months. Truth be told, most of us eat many of the same foods day after day, so once you do the calculations a few times, you'll get a pretty good picture of where you're at.

> Meals are supposed to be nourishment, not a calculation.

A couple of the people on the test panel told me that the thought of putting numbers on their food really leaves them cold. Meals are supposed

---

Leslie's Lessons: "When you cut 200 to 300 calories, you hardly notice it. When you get up to 500 calories, you can get a little hungry and a little cranky. It's a more drastic change. You're trying to find an eating plan and schedule you can live with. If you're cutting 200 calories from your eating and also exercising more, that's a more livable equation for many people than cutting 500 calories per day."

---

to be nourishment, not a calculation. "I know people who have counted calories," panelist Amy N., 24, said to me. "Then they switch to Weight Watchers and they end up counting food points. The people didn't do it in what seemed like a healthy way to me. When I became aware of people counting calories, I just thought, *Oof, I'm not sure that's a good idea.*"

Look, we get it. We all know someone who has become competitive or obsessive with the numbers, and then we've watched as they've gone the other way, eating too little. But the numbers give you a point of reference, a way to be knowledgeable about what you're taking in. You don't have to count calories for the rest of your life.

Being the nosy person that I am, I decided to ring up the calorie total in Leslie's food log from Chapter 2. (Remember, Leslie runs 5 or 6 days, about 20 miles total, a week.)

FOOD	AMOUNT	CALORIES
Pear	1 medium	90
Greek yogurt, vanilla	6 oz	120
Bran Buds	¼ cup	66
Almonds	2 Tbsp	130
Coffee, black	12 oz	0
Almond/raisin mix	⅓ cup	150
Hummus	⅓ cup	135
Feta	¼ cup	100
Whole wheat pita	1 regular size	160
Tomato slices, thick	2	10
Pickle	1 spear	5
Apple, medium	1	95
Cheddar cheese	2 oz	225
Pretzel nuggets	10	100
Grilled salmon	5 oz	350
Salad with mixed greens, peppers, cucumbers, olives, mushrooms, and ¼ cup chopped fruit	3 cups	110
Olive oil vinaigrette	1 Tbsp	80
Wine	5 oz	127
	TOTAL	**2,053**

If you're reluctant to count, know this: As you start to focus on getting enough protein and fruits and vegetables into the mix, you'll find you don't have to worry so much about the calorie total. We'll show you how to tinker with healthy substitutions and get more nutrient bang for your caloric buck in the next few chapters. If you know how to eat the right way, the calorie total naturally falls into line.

Leslie's Lessons: "The idea here is the initial accountability, giving people a point of awareness. I think if people are truly making an investment in trying to make their bodies healthier and trying to lose weight, you can't do that by being clueless. You have to invest some time to at least know the numbers. You do what you want with that, but at least you're informed."

ROXY, 49

Job: Administrative secretary at a hospital pathology department; mother of one

Goals: Lose weight, increase metabolism, and increase speed

Starting weight: 209 pounds

Ending weight: 193 pounds

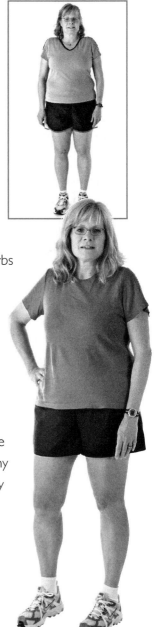

How I Got Here: I got up over 200 pounds and just figured that's where I was going to be at my age. Also, I'd get up early, but I wouldn't eat for a few hours. When I did eat, it was way too many carbs and not enough protein.

What Worked: Adding protein and eating closer to when I woke up instead of waiting until I got to work. Rather than a bagel with cream cheese every day, I made oatmeal at home and added a little protein powder. If I had my bagel, I had it with a single slice of low-fat cheese. Either way, I was full until lunch. Now I make an effort to put canned tuna or chicken on top of my lunchtime salad. The extra protein fills me up for my run later.

Claiming "Me Time": When you're younger and you get married, you always try to make everything perfect. Like your house has to be spotless. Now I don't care if I don't dust the bedroom. I'll straighten up a little bit, but I don't do a major overhaul, so I still have time for exercise. This is for me.

Is It Hunger or Something Else? Sometimes my hunger is from boredom or stress. Feeling overwhelmed can put me in a haze, and I don't realize what I am eating. I try to write in my journal on the days that are very challenging.

Just Move: I try to get some kind of exercise every day, whether it's mowing the grass, going for a walk, or running.

Secret Weapons: I got a Garmin Forerunner 205. What a great tool! It shows your distance, time, and pace. When I see it's getting toward 12-minute-mile pace, I step it up a little. I finished a 5-K race in 33:34. I was so happy!

Chapter 5

The Race
Is On!

Really want to jump-start your motivation? Sign up for a race.

That's right, you. You can enter a race. Sure! Why not?

Don't sign up for one happening this weekend. It shouldn't be next weekend, either. It could be a month from now or 4 months or even a year, but start scouting. Pick a 5-K (which is 3.1 miles) and get it on your calendar.

You can enter a race. Sure! Why not?

Check to make sure at least 500 people enter it, and if you can find one with north of 1,000 entrants, that's even better. The more runners, the merrier. When you have a lot of people around you, you can guarantee that someone will be slower than you. Someone will be walking the whole way. Because that's the number-one fear of every person who enters a race for the first time: *What if I'm last?* Trust us. If you pick a big enough race and you run even just a few minutes of it, you will not be last.

When you find a 5-K that raises money for a cause you believe in, like cancer research or the local Boys & Girls Club, there's even more to like. That way you'll know your race entry fee is going to a worthy cause.

When that race is on your calendar, suddenly you're more focused in your training. You'll keep pushing to see what you can do instead of finding a comfortable level and coasting along for a few weeks. After all, you have a deadline to meet—a race. Also, you'll find even more impetus to get out of bed and train. You don't want to try to fake it through a 5-K when you have a bib number pinned to your shirt. You might even discover that when you're "in training," you treat yourself better. You get more sleep, pass on the ice cream, and stretch a few minutes after a run. Great stuff.

Nola, one of our test panelists, is 42 years old. A few weeks into training, she signed up for a local women's 5-K. She diligently trained for the next 8 weeks and then did the race. Here's the e-mail she sent me afterward:

The race was a great accomplishment for me. I am very proud of it.

Originally my goal was to be able to cross the finish line of the 5-K on June 12 alive. Seriously, as long as I was breathing when I was done, I would be happy—just to be able to do some walking and some running and to say I actually did a 5-K. . . . It would be a check on the ol' bucket list.

But something happened on the way to the 5-K, over the weeks of the program. I slowly set mini goals, and maybe it was the competition of the day, but because it was not hot and sunny (although it was humid), I decided that I really wanted to be able to "run" the whole 5-K—get through it at a jog/run, without doing any walking. That was my new goal. Even if my jogging was slower than some people's walking, that would be fine. I was nervous, though.

Of course, my first mile of the race was 11 minutes and 15 seconds, but I guess I kind of had the adrenaline of the start in me—and I had to slow down a bit after that. I knew my husband and kids were there, waiting at the finish line with a big sign, so that really made me motivated to go quickly at the end of the race. I finished in 37:01, 178th out of 320. The end was an odd sensation . . . the adrenaline that kicked in right when I could see the finish line ahead . . . a whoosh of power that was almost dizzying . . . and I did it; I ran a 5-K! Woo-hoo!

Nola :)

Seriously, if you can't smile after seeing an e-mail like that, you're a running Grinch. Can't you just tell that Nola is going to be carrying that accomplishment around with her, like some invisible charm bracelet?

Finishing a race will be great for you, too. Of course you don't have to run the whole way, but just being in an organized athletic event can change the way you view yourself. You'll see how much fun it is to be a participant, not on the sidelines because you're carrying around too many extra pounds or get winded too easily. It's a major high.

Here's how Amy N. describes running and racing. "I hit high school, and everyone else who was in sports had been in sports for years," she says. "I figured I'd missed that boat forever. But running is open to anyone who wants to try it. The running community is a friendly, encouraging one. I've only ever seen people who are happy when you show up; they're happy that you're there, they don't care that you're slow. They'll cheer you on."

CELEBRITY RUN-INS!

Here's one bonus: If you're in a big urban race, there might be an elite field. You might even be in the same race as an Olympian or two. How's that for a rush? Running is the only sport where the masses get to compete in the same event with the world's best. Sure, you might play pickup basketball, but you're never going to be on the court with LeBron James. Yes, you and your friend play in a tennis league, but you're never going to hit with Maria Sharapova. But if you enter the right race, you might just be behind some international running stars. And that's really cool.

I run the Mini 10-K every year in New York's Central Park. It's a women-only event that draws several thousand runners. In June 2010 I was running along, and who should I come up behind but Paula Radcliffe! She is the women's world record holder in the marathon and hails from Great Britain.

Now, for the record, she was 5 months' pregnant.

She was running the race on a lark, waving to the crowd cheering her on. But hey, I had my brush with an Olympian. You really can't say that about any other sport.

Chat up some friends who are runners. Get their suggestions on fun races. Then sign up and enjoy the experience. Still not convinced? Go watch a race. Seriously, find a 5-K and stand near the finish line until everyone has finished. You'll be surprised at what you see out there: the mix of people, some running, some walking, all having fun.

NOLA, 42

Job: Entrepreneur; mother of two daughters

Goals: Strengthen and tone my body and stay
injury-free

Starting weight: 174 pounds

Ending weight: 163 pounds

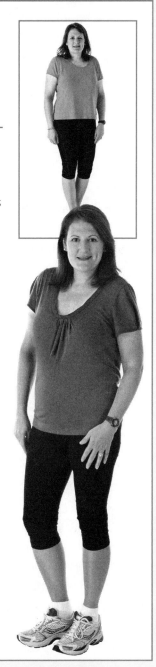

What Worked the Most: I tried the breads that have 5 grams of fiber in them, and I liked them. Running makes me hungrier, but in a good way. I'll be starving after a run, but I don't grab a quick, junky bar. I'll go for something healthier, like fruit. Or lean protein.

Wow! Moment: I was touring Philadelphia with my kids one day last summer. It was 96 degrees, and there was a bit of a walk between museums. They were exhausted and complaining. Had I not been involved in the running program, I would have complained, too. It was really cool to think, *This is nothing, as far as distance goes, and we're just walking, not running. I can SO do this.*

Family Ties: A friend snapped a picture of my two girls holding a sign for me at the end of a 5-K I ran. I love looking at the photo because it's clear on their faces how excited they are for me.

WHO'S HOLDING YOU ACCOUNTABLE?

Signing up for a race is great because you have an event to finish, and you've decided you're going to get yourself in shape to complete it. By paying the entry fee, you've made yourself more accountable in your training.

Other people find different checks and balances to keep them on the way to their goals. Tammy from our test panel weighs herself every morning, first thing. Though experts recommend you only weigh yourself once a week, Tammy can't help it. "I like to know where I am for the day," she says. And her husband, lying in bed, can hear the beep-beep of the bathroom scale. When Tammy emerges from the bathroom, he sticks his hand out of bed for a high five. "Sometimes I go and give him a high five," she says. "Other days I say, 'Nooo! I can't high-five you today!'"

Leslie would probably cringe at Tammy's daily weigh-ins, because a fluctuation of $\frac{1}{2}$ pound here or there can be water weight, not necessarily an accurate indicator of her body fat. But her story strikes a nerve with me. She has her husband on her weight-loss team, and when there's someone else involved to celebrate the successes and urge you on through the rough spots, you're so much more likely to achieve the goal you set.

Here's what a lot of test panelists found: Having *RYBO* to answer to made them a lot more willing to work out and watch their diets. When they realized I'd be e-mailing them or calling them and asking them for their weight every week, it motivated them to get out there—which, they admitted, they might not have done so religiously on their own.

So what's the lesson here? Well, you have to find some way to be accountable in your training. A few people are internally motivated, and that's amazing. They set their minds to doing something and they do it.

The rest of us need the carrot or the stick. Or both. We need someone or something watching over us, nagging us, cajoling us into being our best selves.

> You have to find some way to be accountable in your training.

Maybe we need the support of an anonymous online community offering encouragement.

Think for a moment about what kind of person you are. Are you 100 percent internally motivated? If not, how can you go about developing a support system for yourself? Think about friends you can recruit to join you in becoming a runner. Or just tell a few people about your goals, because you'd better believe they're going to ask you about them. And that's what you want. "At heart, we're all pleasers," Leslie says. "We don't like to let others down, and we don't like to let ourselves down."

Noel Carol, a 57-year-old grandmother on our test panel, started a blog in which she chronicled her workouts. Her friends read it, encouraged her, and became motivated themselves. "I'm so happy that my changes in eating habits have had a positive effect on my family," she says. "My grandson now passes on chips in favor of cantaloupe and carrot sticks. And I know of seven friends who read my blog and have changed their eating and exercise habits."

As Noel Carol proves, the accountability goes both ways.

STAGE 5 WORKOUT

- Walk for 2 minutes 30 seconds. Run for 5 minutes.

- Repeat that sequence three more times.

- End with 3 minutes of walking.

Total workout time: 33 minutes, 20 of which are running.

Do this workout at least three or four times in a week
before moving on to the next stage.

This is a pivotal week. What's going on in this workout? Well, as you're doing every week, you're increasing the run segment. And 5 minutes is a long time to run without stopping. This workout asks you to do that four times. So, at the risk of sounding redundant, you'll have to approach the run very slowly. You want to be able to get through all four running segments, so you can't go charging out of the gate for the first one and quit after two. Pace yourself.

Also, the walking portion decreases this week. If you're pushing too hard during the 5 minutes of running, those 150 seconds of walking are going to feel like they're over before you've had a chance to catch your breath. So keep the run controlled, really slow down on the walk, and see how it goes.

> Keep the run controlled. Pace yourself.

BUILDING A FIRM FOUNDATION

Assuming you've accomplished three or four Stage 4 workouts in a week, you can go ahead and try this one. Remember, it's fine to mix and match in a week. Perhaps you want to do two Stage 4s and two Stage 5s this week. That's fine. You're not locked into anything. You just want to be able to do at least three, preferably four, Stage 5s in a single week before you go on to the workout in the next chapter.

The workout in each stage sets the foundation for the next level of running. It's important to understand that you can't expect to finish the running workouts later in the program if you haven't mastered the earlier ones. Each day that you exercise, you're improving your muscle strength, heart strength, and lung capacity, and you're burning a few hundred extra calories. You don't want to skimp early on.

Also, if you do just one workout each week, it's not really going to help you get in shape. Two workouts per week won't do much, either. Three or four? Now we're talking. It's the habit, the consecutive weeks of walking and running at least every other day, that will show you the results you're seeking.

> Each day that you exercise, you're improving your muscle strength, heart strength, and lung capacity, and you're burning a few hundred extra calories.

ABOUT THOSE SHOES AGAIN

Back in Chapter 2, we said you didn't have to rush out and buy new running shoes unless you really wanted to. Well, now that you're running 20 minutes in a single workout and as much as 1 hour 20 minutes per week, it's a good idea to get running-specific shoes.

Do yourself a favor. For your first pair, skip going to Kohl's or Modell's or ordering online. Instead, find a specialty running store. These are the places like Super Runners Shop in New York City or Fleet Feet in Baltimore or Blue Mile in Indianapolis. If you don't know of one, Google "running store" and your city's name and see what comes up.

The folks who staff these stores are runners. They know what they're looking at when they look at runners' feet. You can tell them how much you're running now, what you hope to accomplish, and about any aches and pains that you have. They'll watch you walk in your socks and be able to tell if you pronate (feet roll in) or supinate (feet roll out) or anything else. Then they'll put you in the right pair of shoes for *your* body. They'll let you jog up and down the street a bit or around the block to see how the shoes feel. Be honest. If they don't fit right, keep trying. You don't get that kind of service at other stores. It's worth it.

Once you've found a pair that you love, you can probably save yourself a few bucks by ordering subsequent pairs online. But you might find yourself returning to the running store for future pairs anyway, because these places are great hubs for beginners. They usually offer group runs for athletes of all abilities. You might be able to pick up a running buddy or two or see some races advertised that you didn't know about.

Shop It!

When I worked in New York City, every time it was a coworker's birthday, we'd celebrate with a giant ice cream cake from Carvel or one of those communal chocolate chip cookies with frosting that's the size of a large pizza, from which everyone slices off a generous serving. A salesperson inked a new contract or someone earned a promotion? Off for beers we went. Many offices, like accounting firms during tax season, bring in food for employees during the busy times so they don't have to leave their desks and stop working to eat.

So let's see: sitting all day in front of a computer, food at arm's length, high-stress environment. . . . Yes, work, in many cases, is making us fat.

Of course *you* decide what goes into your mouth. Leslie likes to remind me when I tell her of an unhealthy day of eating, "Last time I checked, food was an inert object. It doesn't just fly up and settle in your mouth." We're not force-fed, at the office or anywhere else. If we train our brains and learn to anticipate trouble situations, we'll be better able to steer clear.

SUPERMARKET STRATEGIES

Now that I work at home and don't have the temptations of cubicle life at arm's reach, the weekly trip to the grocery store is where I can do the greatest good—or the greatest damage. Every time you step into a supermarket, you're setting yourself up for success or sabotaging your goals.

Let's see how that trip should go.

What's for Dinner?

The most important strategy for conquering the supermarket is having a detailed list. In order to do that, you need to have an idea of what you're serving yourself and your family throughout the week. That doesn't mean you have to be rigid about your menu if you get held up at work or there's a heat wave and you don't feel like eating stew after all. But you should have a sense of the next 7 days: Who is at home, who is traveling for work, who has an evening practice? When do you have time for a more elaborate meal? Which day will you need something quick and easy on the table pronto? When will you have leftovers? A little planning up front will keep you from calling for high-calorie takeout.

Here, Leslie offers suggestions for seven meals in a week. We don't know how big your family is, whether you're one person or eight sitting down to a meal. But we're trying to get your wheels turning.

Sunday: Marinate a skirt steak for 1 hour in a light red wine vinaigrette. (Many brands, including Kraft and Wishbone, make these marinades.) Broil for 5 to 7 minutes per side and cut in thin slices across the grain. Serve with homemade brown rice pilaf: Cook brown rice in chicken broth and add in golden raisins and finely chopped pecans. For a vegetable, roast asparagus. Lay it on a cookie sheet, drizzle with a little olive oil, and sprinkle with sea salt and pepper. Roast at 450°F for 5 to 7 minutes.

Monday: Leftovers: Slice the remaining skirt steak and wrap it in a whole wheat tortilla with pepper strips. Top with jarred salsa.

Tuesday: Roast a chicken with sweet potatoes, or buy a roasted chicken and a side of veggies. Eat half of the chicken with the sweet potatoes or the veggies.

Wednesday: Chop the remaining half roast chicken into bite-size pieces. Cook half a box of rigatoni and a 10-ounce bag of frozen Italian vegetables. Combine with the chicken. Divide the mixture in half again. Top one half with spaghetti sauce and serve hot for today's dinner. Refrigerate the other half.

Thursday: Combine the other half of the chicken-pasta-vegetables with a can of drained cannellini beans and toss in a light vinaigrette dressing. Serve as a pasta salad.

Friday: Grill night. Cut a baking potato into quarters or eighths, toss lightly with olive oil and sea salt, and grill on a piece of foil for about 30 minutes. Skewer chunks of beef, which you can buy precut or cut yourself into approximate 2-inch squares, and grill them, usually about 10 minutes. Assemble other skewers of eggplant, onion, and peppers and grill them alongside the potatoes and meat.

Saturday: Take a pouch of Uncle Ben's whole grain brown "ready rice" and heat in the microwave for 90 seconds. Place the rice in a bowl and top it with mixed greens or baby spinach. Add defrosted frozen, cooked shrimp, or leftover chicken. Top with fresh or canned chunk pineapple packed in water and dress with a sesame vinaigrette.

Bonus meal! Take a fish like cod or roughy, and top with sliced onions and a can of seasoned diced tomatoes. Bake at 375°F until the fish flakes easily with a fork, about 15 minutes. Serve with couscous or quinoa and a side salad.

These meals might not land you on the Food Network, but they're tasty, healthy, fast, and easy. More important, they'll save you a trip to the Chinese restaurant for deep-fried General Tsao's chicken and egg rolls.

Back to the Supermarket

From a meal plan like the one Leslie offers, you can make a detailed list of the meat, veggies, and starches you'll need for dinner. After that you can fill in the foods you'll want to have on hand for breakfast, lunch, and snacks.

The list is your best friend. It saves you money because it keeps you from buying things you already have plenty of. And it makes it easier to resist those two-for-one offers on cookies you're confronted with at the entrance to the store. If something's on your list, you buy it. If it's not, you don't buy it.

> Fifteen minutes spent on your list up front will save you a lot of time, annoyance, and, we dare say, calories later.

The list also saves you time. Honestly, if you've got a few free minutes in your week, do you relish the chance to go back to the supermarket? No! Take a few moments to compile your list and check to see if you need that can of tomatoes or if you already have three of them in your pantry, hidden behind the pasta. Then you won't be running back to the store on multiple occasions during the week. Fifteen minutes spent on your list up front will save you a lot of time, annoyance, and, we dare say, calories later.

Loading Up the Cart

When you shop for weight loss, your cart should have a definite look to it. And Little Debbie snacks aren't part of that look.

- Pick up plenty of produce. Sure, fresh is great, but frozen or canned is also fine, especially if you're going to the store only once a week. You'll eat up the fresh first, then use the frozen and canned later in the week. (Put any fresh produce in the top part of your cart, so the juices from the meat you buy later don't drip down onto it and so it doesn't get squashed.)

Leslie's Lessons: "If you've got all those things in there—produce, dairy, lean meat, whole grains—then the Cheetos and licorice and soda become the top-off instead of the major component. There just isn't room in the cart for the bad stuff."

- Got dairy? Milk should be 1% or fat-free, and yogurt, cottage cheese, and cheese should be low-fat, too.

- Look for lean meats, without a lot of white streaks of fat, and skinless poultry or poultry with easily removed skin. Fish is a healthy choice as long as it's not breaded.

- Breads and cereals should be whole grain and high in fiber. Four brands of bread currently offer 5 grams of fiber per slice: Arnold, Pepperidge Farm, Bran'ola, and Country Hearth. Again, do the flip-and-read to see what you're buying.

- With the exception of milk, almost everything in your cart should be solids. If you're buying juice, make sure it's 100 percent and limit yourself to 4 to 6 ounces daily.

In other words, the foods in your cart should be nutrient rich. "Nutrient rich" is a favorite catchphrase these days among dietitians like Leslie; there's even a Nutrient Rich Foods Coalition set up to educate Americans about the foods that give us the most vitamins and minerals for the fewest calories. High-fiber bread packs more nutritional punch than a handful of fat-free pretzels. (Those pretzels may be fat free, but they're not calorie-free, and what nutrients does your body gain by eating them? A few measly grams of carbohydrate, which none of us are short on to start with.) For a kick-butt shopping list, see what's posted at nutrientrichfoods.org.

CLEAR THE CABINETS

If you have a lot of stuff that doesn't exactly qualify as nutrient rich in your kitchen or desk drawer at work, it's a good time to do a purge. Out with the chips, the full-fat ice cream, the cookies, the Tombstone pizza, the leftover mac 'n' cheese that Aunt Myrtle makes, the Halloween candy that you won't let your kids eat (but that you don't mind sneaking a piece of here and there). Gone.

Leslie's Lessons: "I was looking at the food logs of the people on the test panel right after Easter. They honestly reported what they ate: M&M's, candy, chocolate bunnies. And they told me, 'I ate it because it was there.' Well, if it's there, it's going to get eaten. If it isn't there, we're less likely to leave our house to look for it. Get out the garbage bag and toss in the goodies."

If you don't want to waste food, give it to a family that isn't watching their calorie intake. Or put it in an opaque container in the pantry, out of sight. Or freeze it. You want to create an environment for yourself that's conducive to eating success. If you've got all those temptations around, it gets really, really hard to avoid them.

So start with a kitchen makeover. Get rid of the visual stimuli that might prompt you to overeat. You're full after a meal, but you see the chocolate bunny. It looks good, so you eat it.

No longer. Not in your house.

Just by cutting down the amount of treats you consume, you can easily slice several hundred calories per week from your total. And that is what you want: the number of calories going in the mouth to head south, the number of calories burned through exercise to head north. That's the essence of *RYBO*.

TAMMY, 43

Job: IT specialist

Goals: To lose weight and become faster

Starting weight: 210 pounds

Ending weight: 199 pounds

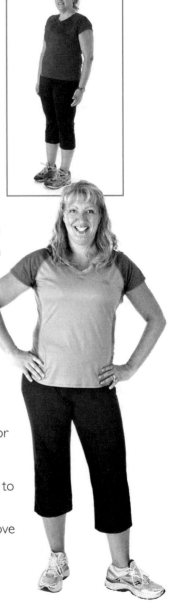

A Roller Coaster: I've always been big. And I was a smoker from the time I was 15 until I was 36. My highest weight was 229. I was totally disgusted with myself.

In 2007 I got married, I started running, and I was down to 160. I felt fabulous and I looked great. Then I came down with mono. I had to sleep a lot, plus I ate a lot and had no activity, and I gained a bunch of the weight back.

Work Doesn't Help: I work in IT, so I'm sitting on my butt all day, and often I'm making long drives between sites. I try to go out during the day and walk in the parking lot. When I can't go outside, I'll do two flights of stairs in the office, five or six times in a row. That gets my heart rate up.

Friends on the Run: I have a group of ladies I like to run with on Saturday mornings. They get me out there, even if these days I'm trailing behind them. I love to be able to talk while I'm running.

Be Accountable: It's helpful for me to have to e-mail my weight to someone every week. I made a spreadsheet to keep track of my workouts. I include everything, like walking the dog and walks I take at work, as well as formal exercise. I use it to record my weight as well as things like if I've been sick and am taking antibiotics or if I'm on vacation. It helps me see how I'm doing and stay active.

The Scale Beckons: I have a bad habit of weighing myself almost every day. I know I'm only supposed to weigh myself once a week, but my scale stares at me every morning and says, "Come on and step on me!" I try not to let the number make me crazy, but I use it to keep myself in check.

Using Technology: The Daily Plate (thedailyplate.com) has a cool application I downloaded for my iPhone. It counts my calories and tracks my fluid intake. It's really user-friendly.

Put Your Company to Work for You: I work for a large insurance business that offers employees free consultations with a nutritionist, so I had a conversation with her. Why not? She was really helpful. People should take advantage of the benefits their employers pay for.

Chapter 6

A Jog, Not a Sprint

Our test panelist Becky discovered that she loves running. Absolutely loves it. She joined First Strides, the local running program for women, and entered 14 races in her first 18 months as a runner. Now she does about a 13-minute-mile pace—and can't get enough.

"I feel great when I run," she says. "I think how fortunate I am that my body is able to do this. At first it was very hard and I thought, *No way.* But then one night a First Strides mentor said to me, 'You are trying too hard and tiring yourself out. Slow down; take smaller steps.' And boom, just like that I could last longer. It was doable. Every week as the program progressed, I would be thinking, *Yikes!* And then when I would do it, I was thinking, *Wow!*"

Becky started running when she was 51, after she had been treated for colon cancer. It was the first time in her life that she had been involved in an organized sport. And when you're wearing cancer-colored glasses, your perspective gets a total makeover. While many beginning runners might dwell on the discomfort, not Becky. "After having cancer, running makes me think of life, not death," she says. The First Strides organizers loved her attitude so much that they asked her to be a mentor for the next class of women learning how to run.

She and her running friends posted pictures on Facebook weekly, every time they increased the amount of running they did. "Sometimes I'd be on the way home from a run and I'd feel like I could stop the car and do the whole thing again," she says.

Clearly, Becky is hooked on exercise. Are you hooked on exercise yet? You know, the feeling that your day isn't complete without a good sweat? That a challenging workout (but one you can finish) greases the skids and makes everything go a little smoother? If you've caught the exercise bug, then you'll recognize the feeling I'm talking about.

Are you hooked on exercise?

For a while—a long time, it seems—we only appreciate exercise when it's over. We feel virtuous for having done it, and we're glad we pushed ourselves out the door. Whew. Check that off the day's to-do list.

But there comes a point when the actual "during" portion of exercise isn't so bad, either. You're out there and you start running, and it feels much easier than you anticipated it would before you started. You feel like you've got a good stride going. In fact, it's downright invigorating. It goes by quickly, and you're sort of sorry it has to end.

Not there yet? Trust me. It will happen.

You've probably heard people talking about endorphins causing the famous "runner's high." Scientists debate the role of endorphins; some think anandamide, another chemical the body produces that the brain feasts on, might be the cause. Whatever the body chemistry reason, many people experience a sense of well-being during and after a run. For some it's a mild sensation. For others it's more intense.

Becky got the high within a few weeks of starting to run, thanks to the person who noticed her struggling and told her to slow down. For some it can take a lot longer. When I spoke to another test panelist, Stephanie, after the study ended, she was very diplomatic about her thoughts on running. I think she was afraid to hurt my feelings. "Sarah, I never get to a place where I feel like I'm running smoothly," she said. "I feel like it's always an effort."

But then came the "but." "But I was surprised that I could do more than I thought," she told me. Stephanie ran most of the way of a 5-K race, taking only a couple of 30-second walk breaks. She finished in 45:41.

Stephanie dropped 12 pounds in 12 weeks, from 231 to 219. She's pleased with the results, and she attributes them to running. But it's still

Budd's Buzz: "Nonwalkers and nonrunners have this sense of physical exertion being painful. They feel fatigued, and they might feel some discomfort. But the person who has walked or run for a long time? That exertion is ecstasy. We feel like 'Finally! I can get out there and do something physical!'"

not something she relishes when she's out there. That will continue to take time. For now, the results are enough to motivate her to keep at it.

Taking the running portion slowly and building up gradually will minimize the discomfort you'll feel. The hope is that soon enough, you'll cross over from one of those people who can't wait for exercise to end and join the camp of those who can't wait for it to begin.

STAGE 6 WORKOUT

- Walk for 3 minutes. Run for 7 minutes.

- Repeat that sequence two more times.

- End with 3 minutes of walking.

Total workout time: 33 minutes, 21 of which are running.

Do this workout at least three or four times in a week
before moving on to the next stage.

With this workout you're doing more than 20 minutes of running in each session. The walking is down to 12 minutes. Over last week and this week, the balance has completely shifted in favor of running. Give yourself some credit for how far you've come!

Here's the thing: The more you run, the more weight you lose and the easier it is to . . . keep running. It's hard to get the momentum going at first. But once you get on track, consistent, and committed to your workouts, the more calories you'll shed and the less you'll weigh. It takes less effort to pick your feet up and run, and you can go longer. Then you'll get a little faster, go a little farther, and torch even more calories. Plus, your

The more you run, the more weight you lose
and the easier it is to . . . keep running.

heart and lungs are better conditioned already. And when there's less of you to move, they don't have to work quite so hard. You feel better even though you're doing more. It's a happy circle.

 # Attitude Adjustment

Our test panelist Jenn, 27, experienced the quickest weight loss. She lost 16 pounds, going from 212 to 196, in the first 6 weeks of the program. Her results are not typical, Leslie and Budd warn. Most people don't lose weight that fast, nor should they. But shedding the pounds helped her enjoy her workouts more. Here's what she said about doing the Stage 6 workout:

> The first few weeks were difficult, but starting when I was running 7 minutes and walking 3, I noticed that I really don't have to talk myself into running much anymore. I started to feel it more in my muscles, rather than feeling like I was just sucking wind. It started to get easier after I dropped a few pounds.
>
> I think the plan was more of a mental change for me. I was pretty sedentary before I started. From time to time I had halfheartedly committed to other exercise plans. I would start them, then give up after a few sessions of overdoing it without seeing results. The running plan has been nice because it is very gradual and is only a half hour commitment a few times a week. It's almost more difficult to find a reason that I can't work out than it is to just do it!

SEE HOW FAR YOU'VE COME

I guarantee that if you were to go back and do the workout that was 3 minutes of running and 3 minutes of walking, you'd feel like it's a cinch.

That's progress. In fact, it might be a good idea, on a 4th day of running in a week, to go back to doing one of the earlier stage workouts just to see how you feel. So your week might look something like this:

Monday: **Stage 6 workout**

Wednesday: **Stage 6 workout**

Friday: **Stage 6 workout**

Saturday: **Stage 4 workout**

As you breeze through Saturday's workout, I promise that you'll get a sense of the improvement you've made. And you'll probably go a little longer just to feel like you've done a "real" workout. My, how times have changed in just a few weeks!

HOW MANY CALORIES ARE WE TALKING?

Here's a good time to see how the calorie equation changes as the running increases.

Let's go back to that 200-pound person we used as an example in Chapter 2. Back then we assumed that person was covering about 1.7 miles and mostly walking, so we used the walking multiplier, 0.53, multiplied by body weight multiplied by distance. And we came up with 106 calories per mile, so 180 calories burned for that workout. The 160-pound person would have burned 144 calories.

Now here's where the numbers change. I'm assuming, with 21 minutes of running, that a beginning runner is covering 1.5 miles. With 12 minutes of walking, that beginner goes 0.7 mile.

But by this point in the program, the beginner has already lost 5 pounds. That changes the math, too. So let's see how that looks: body weight (195 pounds) × 0.75 (calories burned per mile of running) × 1.5 miles. That figures to be 219 calories.

Now for the walking portion: body weight (195 pounds) × 0.53

(calories burned per mile of walking) × 0.7 (walking distance). That's 72 calories.

Add the two together and we get 291 calories. In 33 minutes. Not bad, eh?

And the 160-pound person, who now weighs 155, burns about 232 calories in the same workout. That's nothing to sneeze at, either.

Remember, these are approximations. If you don't know how far you're going in miles, it's impossible to know your calorie burn. I'm using 14 minutes per mile for running speed and 18 minutes per mile for walking speed. That's pretty conservative. If you're going faster, you're increasing the rate of calorie burning.

So don't get too obsessed with the numbers.

The point is this: Compared to four chapters ago, by upping the running, the first person is burning about 110 extra calories per session. The second runner is burning an additional 88.

DEFICIT SPENDING

Remember the fundamental premise: In order to lose weight, you have to create a calorie deficit. By eating less (or burning more) calories than your body uses in a day, you'll lose pounds and shed fat.

The deficit grows with each mile you run. By doing this Stage 6 workout four times a week, that 195-pound person will have torched 1,164 calories; the 155-pound runner will have burned almost 928 calories. When you get to four-figure calorie expenditures, you'll see results on the scale.

Continue to eat right, too, and the deficit will grow. Deficits are bad for the government, but they're just what you want.

BE SELECTIVE WITH SPORTS DRINKS

The sports drink industry is very clever with its marketing. We've all watched the commercials and gotten the message it's sending. So after you've finished a 33-minute workout, especially on a hot day, you might feel like you need a Gatorade to replace your lost electrolytes.

Don't be tempted.

Sports drinks have a *lot* of calories per bottle. Lemon-lime-flavored Gatorade has 50 calories per 8-ounce serving. But the 20-ounce bottle, which is the one you'd grab at a convenience store, has 2½ servings in it. So if you're really thirsty and chug the whole thing, that would be 125 calories right there.

You can undo a lot of the good you just did in your workout by drinking one of these things.

When you're thirsty, it's important to replace the lost fluids. But good old water will do the trick. Or have milk; at least you'll be getting some protein and calcium, too. Milk is nutrient rich. Sports drinks? Not so much.

FOOD TALK Slow It Down!

Check the clock when you take your first bite of dinner. Look at it again when you're finished eating. How much time has elapsed? Five minutes? Ten? More than that?

The longer, the better. Scientists know that it takes at least 15 to 20 minutes for the nerve endings in the gut to send the signal to the brain that says, "Yup, I'm fed! You can stop eating now!"

We've all had that experience of being really hungry, wolfing down a larger meal than we're used to, and then feeling uncomfortably full after. But even if you overeat by just a little bit at every meal, you accrue a lot of extra calories that your body doesn't need—which you then have to find a way to rid yourself of later.

When you get up to training for a half-marathon or a marathon, and you're routinely completing training runs of an hour and longer, then you can start working a little bit of sports drink into the mix. Skip it for now.

LINGER OVER MEALS

You have to teach yourself to eat slower, simple as that. It can be a gradual process of increasing the amount of time you take for meals. If you're used to taking 3 minutes for breakfast, slow down and take 5,

> You have to teach yourself to eat slower.

then gradually work up to 10. If you consume your lunchtime sandwich in front of your computer in 5 minutes, stretch it out. Eat half, wait for a few minutes, and have a few sips of water or whatever you're drinking. Then eat the other half.

Ultimately, you want to enjoy dinner by stretching the meal out to at least 15 or 20 minutes.

We can anticipate your protest: *First I have to work out three or four times a week, and now you want me to take longer for dinner? I just don't have time!*

Make time for dinner. Dinner has so many benefits, and a lot of them have nothing to do with weight loss. Yes, if you eat slowly, you'll consume fewer calories. But you'll also reconnect with your loved ones. Studies have shown that kids who eat dinner with their parents are smarter and get into less trouble. If you concentrate on dinner, you might actually taste something. You can enjoy the experience of the food in your mouth instead of inhaling it and getting on to the next thing. Dinner is not something you want to check off your to-do list. It should be an enjoyable part of the day, when you linger and savor the experience.

Leslie's Lessons: "I started back to work full-time 6 weeks after both of my boys were born. But my husband and I decided early on it was important to have dinner together as a family. We didn't eat until 8:00 or later, because that's when everyone was available. After school, my kids would come home and eat a substantial snack so they wouldn't be ravenous until 8:00. Any children who have sports in the evening aren't comfortable if they're full of food and running around a field."

YOU HAVE TEETH, SO USE 'EM

The easiest thing you can do to slow down your mealtime is to chew your food. Seriously. It might sound dumb until you try it. Take a bite, put your fork down, and chew your food. Taste it. Savor the flavors and textures. Then swallow. Only then do you pick up your fork again. Instead of tearing off big pieces of food that you gulp down unchewed or sitting there with spoon or fork hovering an inch from your mouth, make a conscious effort to chew and put your utensil down between bites.

Here Leslie shares other tips for making slow dinners a reality.

- Sit down for your meals. Don't eat at the counter.

- Look at your food. Take time to taste it. Be mindful of what's going into your mouth.

- Find a time when you can slow down and focus on feeding yourself. Tune out distractions. Turn off your phone and the TV. This is the time for you to nourish yourself.

- Talk to people. It takes longer to eat when you're talking to someone because it's rude to talk with your mouth full!

- Try to go a whole week without consuming anything in the car. You can't be concentrating on the road and your food at the same time. Two hands on the wheel.

- Eat in like you're eating out. It doesn't cost a cent more to mimic at home what you might get at a restaurant. Put your salad on the table, eat it, and then have the main course. That extends the time it takes you to eat.

- Use the dining room. When the main course is not right there in front of you, it takes a little more time because you have to go to the kitchen for it.

- Avoid family-style. When the food is at arm's length, you're tempted to reach out and eat more than you need. In the morning, measure yourself a bowl of cereal, then put the box away.

- Don't sit in front of the TV with a bag of anything next to you. It's okay if you decide you want a snack at night in front of your favorite show, but measure out a finite amount of food, put it on a plate, and eat it. Don't leave the bag open so you can reach in for a handful every few minutes.

- If you need to eat a bigger snack in the afternoon so you can postpone dinner until everyone has time to sit down together, that's fine. Carve out time to enjoy your food and eat well. Don't try to cram a meal into the 10 minutes between the PTA meeting and your kid's swimming practice.

- You might have to cut back on something else to have time to feed yourself well. If that means 10 fewer minutes on Facebook at night, it's a trade-off well worth making.

Our test panel had some funny things to say about their attempts to eat slowly. "Apparently I don't chew anything," Amy N. told me. Harrison actually made himself eat with chopsticks to slow down. And then there's Dorene's family. We'll let her explain:

> I think eating more slowly was one of the harder aspects of the whole program for my family to adjust to, especially with our spring schedule, because we tend to eat and run. Also, I had not realized how many times I would get up from the table to get something for someone or to take care of this or that.
>
> So we were sitting together eating one night, and between my husband and son, it seemed I was up and down constantly. Well, unfortunately for my husband, he asked for one too many things. In a moment of frustration, which is totally out of character for me, I slammed my fork down on the table and said, "I AM TRYING TO EAT MORE SLOWLY AND TAKE MY TIME WITH THIS MEAL! AND YOU TWO ARE NOT HELPING!"
>
> There was a moment of stunned silence, followed by a sheepish apology from my husband. Then we all laughed at how silly it sounded. But I have gotten to finish more of my meals without interruptions, and I have noticed that eating more slowly and paying attention to when I am full does help, even more so at a restaurant. Several times I have eaten only a portion of what I would have consumed before trying this tip.

RUNNING'S REWARDS: CAN I EVER HAVE A TREAT?

Finish up a good run, push yourself to run for more time than you ever have, and you might feel the urge to reward yourself with food. And it's usually something sweet or higher in fat than is good for you. It's true that sometimes when you're working out more intensely, you do get hungrier. A salad is not going to cut it.

It's a common instinct. When I run a race I'm happy with or slog through a long, slow run for more than 8 or 9 miles, I start dreaming of the chicken tikka masala, drowning in oil, at my favorite Indian restaurant. If that's not in the cards, my mind drifts to the custard at Rita's. Has to be chocolate. A generous portion, thank you very much.

Unfortunately, as we've demonstrated in previous chapters, the "reward" usually exceeds the calorie burn from the exercise. If you're not paying attention, you can undo all the good you've just done.

Budd gets agitated about this. "Food is food, food is fuel," he practically yells. "Food is not a reward!" He suggests getting out of the

Leslie's Lessons: "Put it in perspective. Say to yourself, *I really am hungrier right now.* Then ask: *What do I really feel like eating?* Turn the mind-set around, and get away from the constant denial. *(Oh, I shouldn't, this is bad, what's the matter with me?)* Think about what would be really satisfying, have it, and then move on. *All right, I really don't feel like having my oatmeal today because I did run hard and I would like something indulgent* is more honest than trying to ignore the feeling. That tends to blow up in your face afterward, when you'll completely overeat."

habit of rewarding running with calories in the mouth. Make it something completely different: a new running shirt or watch or pedicure or massage. Create a list of nonfood related items or activities that you consider to be "indulgences" and reward yourself when you've hit your milestones. This will help to keep you motivated without undoing any of your hard work.

> You can learn to have treats in a limited way.

Leslie is a little more understanding. It's human nature to reward ourselves, not punish ourselves. It's what we're programmed to do. The key is to think about what you really want, have it, and be done.

You can learn to have treats in a limited way. "How about a cupcake?" Leslie says. "That's not necessarily terrible in the overall scheme of things. It's having the indulgence, but doing it in a controlled portion. If you really feel like having ice cream in the summer, instead of buying a pint of Ben & Jerry's, go buy a cone. The person behind the counter is in charge of scooping, not you."

THE "I'VE BLOWN IT!" MIND-SET

Though the run/reward cycle can erase the calorie deficit you've worked so hard to achieve, that's not as damaging as the "I've already blown it" mind-set.

Here's how that thinking goes: *I went to a birthday party in the afternoon and I had a big piece of cake with frosting and a flower. So now my day of eating is wrecked and I might as well continue on and have Mexican for dinner with a margarita and ice cream tonight.*

Whoa, whoa, whoa! It's not the cake, which might be a couple of hundred calories, that's the trouble. As Leslie says, we get to wheel and deal with our calories several times a day. So you had the cake? Fine! Later on, skip the roll with your dinner and double up on the veggies, and you'll be okay. No harm, no foul. But this off-to-the-races mentality, that's what sinks us.

Leslie's Lessons: "The problem is never with the initial response, like the first piece of cake or the cookies. It's what happens after that's the problem. People set up such rigid guidelines for themselves. Then it's 'Uh-oh, I deviated, therefore I've blown it, so I might as well continue eating until I go to bed.' You need to get out of the 'I'm good' or 'I'm bad' mind-set. Instead, try saying, 'I feel better because I ate that food. Maybe it was more caloric than I wanted, but it's not the end of the world,' and move on. With that perspective, people will be far more successful with continuing on that path to weight loss."

SECRETS OF THE TEST PANEL

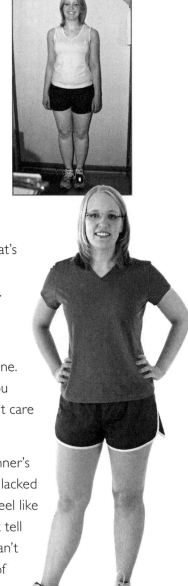

AMY N., 25

Job: Managing editor of a music magazine, *Sing Out!*

Goals: To build up my heart and lungs, offset a
   sedentary lifestyle, burn fat, and build muscle

Starting weight: 144 pounds

Ending weight: 146 pounds

Starting waist: 30 inches

Ending waist: 28¾ inches

Advice for Beginning Runners: You need to
have the mind-set that you're doing something
healthy for yourself, not really for anyone else. That's
how I stuck with it. I've never been a competitive
person. I don't come from an athletic background.
Running is really accessible. It's open to whoever
wants to try it.

The running community is a friendly, encouraging one.
I've only ever seen people who are happy when you
show up, they're happy that you're there, they don't care
that you're slow. They'll cheer you on.

Build Your Confidence: I signed up for a beginner's
running class last year, but after the class ended, I lacked
discipline to continue on my own. But this year I feel like
a runner. It's part of my routine. Before I wouldn't tell
my friends I was running; this year I'll tell them I can't
get together until after I do my run. I'm the kind of

person who likes to learn something well before I tell other people about it.

Race High: I ran my second race ever and finished a minute faster than the last time. I didn't take a single walking break. I found a buddy, and we ran the whole race together, keeping each other accountable and silently pushing each other to keep going. We whipped through the first mile in 10 minutes and hit the 2-mile mark at 21:25, and I crossed the finish line at 34:04.

Forget the Scale: I keep weighing in at a consistent 146. I was hoping maybe it would go down a pound or two. But I feel good. I look at my legs and they amaze me. They carried me 3.1 miles without stopping. How could I not love them?

Ignore the Negative Voice: I have a hard time getting four runs in each week, but I manage it one way or another, even if it means cutting one a little short. It's more of a mental problem than a physical one. When I'm actually out there, it's really not bad at all. But the voice in the back of my head keeps telling me not to push hard or hurt myself or get discouraged. Thanks, voice, but I got this. Really. Have a little faith.

Chapter 7

Fight the Urge to Sit

Throughout the time the test panel was up and running, Noel Carol, 57, was great about sending me feedback. She dutifully sent me her workouts every week. Part exercise log, part travelogue, they were charming to read. Here's a 6-day sample:

5/20: Tried to do workout but only made it through 5-minute warmup, 4-minute run, then stopped, too tired. Walked for 25 minutes at Voorhees in evening (saw my first spring black bear) and did 20 push-ups, 20 sit-ups.

5/21: 6 reps of 1 walk, 4 run on treadmill, plus warmup and cooldown. Incline up to 3 on treadmill. Later walked at Voorhees for 20 minutes.

5/22: Drove 12 hours (6 hours each way) to Pittsburgh and back for niece's baby shower.

5/23: 6 reps of 1 walk, 4 run plus warmup and cooldown.

5/24: Very tired, walked 3 minutes, ran 5 minutes, then stopped.

5/25: Warmup, then 2 reps of 9 running × 2 walking, 2:8×1, plus cooldown. Felt g-r-e-a-t! Walked at Voorhees later 20 minutes+, was a beautiful night!

A bunch of things strike me about Noel's entries. First, a bear? I expected the entry to then make note of a sprint back to the car. But she was unfazed.

Second, Noel provides a lot of information in her log with just a few sentences. You do get a very accurate picture of her physical activity in a day and her energy level at that time. And in some small way, you get a sense of this busy woman's life (full-time state employee, daughter, mother, grandmother) during that period.

Third, she's listening to her body. On the days she starts out for a run and she's dog tired, she stops. Now, I'm sure if a coach like Budd were supervising her closely, he might look at this and encourage her to stop running on those tired days, keep walking for 5 more minutes, then try a few shorter segments of running again. But at least she's not pushing herself to the point of misery, exhaustion, and possible injury. And on the days she feels "g-r-e-a-t," she runs longer. She gets it about being flexible.

The most striking point about Noel's log is that she's active most days—sometimes twice a day. She's frequently doing 20-minute walks in the evening. And unless she's in the car for 12 hours, she's attempting some form of exercise daily.

MOVE IT!

This is important. If you want to give the scale a nudge in the downward direction, work more movement into your day outside of your formal workouts. Walk at lunch, walk the dogs, walk the kids. Go for a bike ride after dinner, do some gardening. Stand up during phone calls. When you're watching your child's soccer game, leave the lawn chair at home and try walking up and down the sideline. Every little bit helps.

We've all heard the point about parking farther away at the store; turns out, this really is good advice. It drives me crazy to see people circling a parking lot looking for a spot close to the door. They burn all that gas but no extra calories. Turn into the parking lot, pull into the first space you come to, and get out of the car!

Anytime you can get off your butt and move—even if it's not to run but just to stroll—it's better than the alternative: sitting. I am lucky that I

> If you want to give the scale a nudge in the downward direction, work more movement into your day outside of your formal workouts.

have a little ledge in my home office. I've written a fair portion of this book standing up. I stick my computer on top of a phonebook on that ledge and it's the right height for me. Simply standing up for 15 minutes at a time helps me focus on the task and maybe think a little differently. And then I'll return to my chair, where I'm now painfully aware that my calorie-burning rate is a measly 56 per hour.

A 2009 book, *Move a Little, Lose a Lot,* by James Levine, MD, a doctor at the Mayo Clinic, made it clear just how much movement has been engineered *out* of our days. We get up, we sit in the car on the way to work, we sit at our desks for 8 hours, we drive home, we sit for dinner, we head for the couch. That kind of lifestyle does nothing to move the BMR beyond the sedentary rate we talked about back in Chapter 1. (Dr. Levine, by the way, attempts to engineer movement back into his days by mounting his desk over a treadmill. He walks on it at 1 mph while he works.)

Remember the weight-loss truth we hold to be self-evident: To lose weight, you need to create a calorie deficit. And doing four workouts, each burning 300 calories, goes a long way. If you've never been active before, you'll see results right away. But if you can burn a few extra calories in the morning, some midday, a few more at night—by taking the stairs, walking across a long parking lot, taking a walk with a friend instead of going out to eat—you'll help add to your total in the "calories burned" category. Believe me, your fat doesn't care if you burn the calories when you're wearing running shoes and an iPod or heels or a tie.

I used to live on the Upper East Side of Manhattan, between First and York Avenues. Every morning I had to walk 3½ wide blocks—close to ½ mile—to the subway on Lexington Avenue. Same thing on the return. That was before I did any formal exercise. These days I pull my car into the driveway, press the automatic garage door opener, and take about four steps into the house. No wonder I've fought the creep of the pounds since I moved to the 'burbs. And, incidentally, when I return to Manhattan for meetings, I'm surprised by how tired my feet and legs feel after all the walking.

JUNE, 31

Job: Accounting paraprofessional

Goal: To run an entire 5-K

Starting weight: 198 pounds

Ending weight: 184 pounds

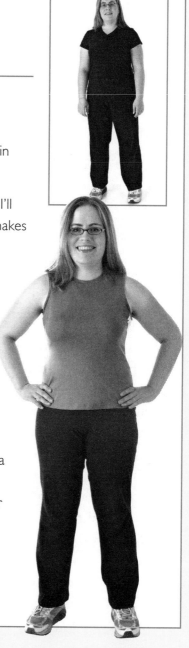

Wow! Moment: I finished my first 5-K in 44:15!

How to Get Out There: I tell myself I'll feel better once I get started. Running makes me feel more emotionally balanced. It helps me pull my head out of the clouds or use up extra energy on a hyperactive day.

What Worked the Most: Keeping a food log. I can't remember what I've eaten unless I write it down. With a log, I can see that my eating is balanced.

Avoiding Diet Pitfalls: Once I got into a routine of eating healthfully, if I cheated, I would notice how badly I felt. I remember that now when I am tempted.

Convinced? Good. Take a page out of Noel's log and try to be active on most days. In fact, take a moment to write down three times where you can add a little more movement to your day.

_____

_____

_____

Here are mine:

Park the car at the bottom of our driveway and walk up to the house at least once a day.

Add 15 more minutes of standing computer time per day until I get to 1 hour.

Race the kids around the house three times before dinner.

NOT-SO-PERFECT DAYS

So you're on your way out the door, gym bag over your shoulder, when your boss stops you to ask for an update on the new client pitch you're making Friday. Or you're stuck in traffic on the way to the park and the minutes are just ticking away. Instead of 30 minutes until you have to pick your son up at swim practice, it's now 23 . . . 22 . . . 21 . . .

What do you do? Work out or bag it?

Get going. Twenty minutes is better than 15, 15 is better than 10. Do whatever you can in that space. A workout that's cut short is so much better than no workout at all, and you'll feel less frustration that night, too.

The reverse of that, busy runners know, is sometimes you have to call an audible. If the boss can't be placated in 5 minutes, you don't want to lose your job over a run. When the weather is hurricane-like, stay home and pop in an exercise DVD. Run tomorrow. There's a line between healthy commitment and obsession.

Reminder: Protect Your Workout

Ultimately, you have to be stubborn about your running. It is *your* time. Yes, some conflicts are unavoidable. If you can convince yourself to work out first thing in the morning, the number of possible infringements on your time is fewer.

Roxy, one of our test panelists, had a revelation one spring day after she started running: "If my husband can devote so much time to improving his golf game, why can't I get out there for my running? He practices, so why can't I?" Excellent point, Roxy. Of course she has other things taking up her time: her job in a hospital pathology department; volunteer work with her local fire company; and spending time with family, neighbors, and friends.

But she sat her husband down and said, essentially, she was not cleaning the house to perfection anymore, and if they were out of milk, her husband or son could get it. She was going to get her running in. "I have to take some time for myself," she said. "Things aren't always going to be perfect, but that's the way it's going to be."

And you know what? Her husband didn't protest at all. He loves her, and he understands she needs this.

I wish I had been a fly on the wall for that conversation. Roxy, by the way, went from 209 pounds at the start of our test period to 193 in 12 weeks. "This is the first part of my journey, and I lost 3 inches off my waist, which I will take with pride!" she says.

Trust me. It's okay to be selfish about your workout. You might feel guilty at first, but who knows? You could also discover you're a better spouse, parent, friend, or employee during the other 23½ hours of the day if you take ½ hour for yourself. Get the word out: Your exercise time is for you, and there had better be a darn good reason for anyone to interrupt you.

STAGE 7 WORKOUT

- Walk for 2 minutes. Run for 8 minutes.

- Repeat that sequence two more times.

- End with 3 minutes of walking.

Total workout time: 33 minutes, 24 of which are running.

Do this workout at least three or four times
in a week before moving on to the next stage.

I hate to break this to you: From this point forward, the most walking that you get to do between running segments is 2 minutes. Yes, a mere 120 seconds. Doesn't feel like much. But remember, you asked for it! You wanted to become a runner, right?

I'm about to say again what I've written several times before. You have to go slow on the run and slower on the walk. At the end of 8 minutes of running, you should not be gasping for breath. In fact, you should feel like you could continue running if you needed to. That's the most important part of this program: going slowly enough to be successful.

If you're still breathing hard, try to shorten your stride and slow your speed so you're not going any faster than a brisk walk. There are no time trials and no deadlines in this book.

Hang out with this workout for a few weeks if you need to—however long it takes until you get comfortable with it. It isn't really that different from the Stage 6 workout; you're only shifting 1 minute at a time from the walking side to the running side. But excluding the cooldown, you're up to 75 percent running with this stage, which is a long way from where you started.

ACHES AND PAINS

Our test panel held up remarkably well through their first 12 weeks of running. In fact, many reported they felt better, and the feet and shin and knee tenderness they worried about at the beginning of the program didn't bother them at all. They were going slowly enough and losing weight, so running went a long way toward eradicating some of the chronic achiness they felt when they were heavier and not moving as much.

If you're doing everything as Budd prescribes—building up gradually, taking it slowly, trying to give yourself a day off between most workouts, wearing supportive shoes—you should be good to keep going. But if you find yourself with new pain, ask yourself a few questions.

Are you tired or hurt? Tired is not a bad thing, and sometimes when you get yourself out the door, you feel completely revitalized a few minutes later. If the flattened-by-a-steamroller feeling doesn't dissipate after 10 or 15 minutes, bag it and try tomorrow.

When it's pain, is it running-related pain? Is it new? Does it get worse with running? Proceed with caution if the answer to any of these questions is yes. Usually, the garden-variety getting-into-shape twinges ease during the off day after a run. If they don't, give yourself an additional day or two off. If you still feel a sharp pain on the 4th day after a run, that's when it's time to call a doctor. Look for a sports medicine specialist who runs.

Budd's Buzz: "You are the best judge of how you feel. Don't keep pushing through an injury just because you want to get that last workout of the week in or you want to do that race. Better to modify your training program with a couple of extra days off or going back to a little more walking, a little less running, than to be completely derailed by an injury. Usually it's the 'just 1 more day' mentality that gets people into trouble. 'Let me do my workout today, and then I'll take some time off.' But by then the damage is done."

RUNNING ETIQUETTE: MY PARTNER IS SLOWING ME DOWN!

Every once in a while, the most committed of running buddies start to diverge in their abilities. And while that might not be so noticeable when you're running for only 2 or 3 minutes at a time, at 8 minutes it becomes obvious.

If you're the slower of the pair, you should encourage your partner to go ahead. This is the right thing to do. You can still meet together for the run, do the first walking portion together, and then start running together. Then you'll separate a bit. When it comes time to walk, the faster partner turns around and walks in the direction of the slower friend. Then when it's time to run again, you'll start together for the next portion. Repeat as needed.

While a running friend can be integral to your success, you don't have to run every step side by side. The running relationship is mutually beneficial in so many other ways: for the motivation on days you don't feel like getting out there, for the friendly face, for the high five at the end, and for the common understanding of what you're trying to accomplish.

Budd's Buzz: "It's always a help if you can plan to meet a friend for a workout. The best thing you can say if you're significantly slower is 'Look, we'll meet, we'll go for the run, but you're faster than I am, so just go ahead. I'm out here, I'm good, and we'll meet up at the finish.'"

ADD ONE RED, YELLOW, ORANGE, GREEN, OR PURPLE FOOD TO *EVERY* MEAL

I checked with Leslie on this, and unfortunately, red wine does not count as adding a color to a meal. Bummer. Lucky Charms, with their different colored marshmallows, don't count, either.

Color It!

Fruits and veggies are loaded with vitamins and minerals your body needs to function, keep your immune system up, and maintain strong bones, muscles, and teeth. They contribute to the liquid our bodies need in a day—about 90 ounces for women, 125 for men—which we'll address later. You have to chew them to eat them, so your mouth is busy and you're eating slower.

Vegetables and fruits also have fiber, which is a big deal for our bodies. Women are supposed to get 25 grams of fiber daily; men need 38. Why is fiber so important? It contributes to making you feel full. That's because it takes longer to leave the stomach and it attracts water to the gut, so you're not hungry again right away after eating high-fiber foods. Also, the body does more work clearing a high-fiber food through your system than it does digesting something that's low in fiber. So fiber burns more calories during digestion without your even realizing it. Experts call this the thermogenic effect of food. To me, the only thing that matters is *See ya, calories.*

Now, you want to be careful when you're adding a lot of fiber to your diet. Add 2 or 3 grams, and stay at that level for a week. Then add a few more. Don't try to go from, say, 12 grams of fiber to 25 in a single day or you'll be doubled over with abdominal cramps. And you might find you need to be careful of the timing. If you eat a lot of fiber before your run, you might experience tummy troubles during your workout.

Leslie often takes the Pitt athletes on field trips to the grocery store. It's an eye-opening experience for them because they're learning how much food costs and how much to buy, and they see the variety of colorful foods available to them that aren't Skittles or Cheetos.

(Leslie once taught the women's basketball players how to choose cantaloupes by shaking and sniffing them. Then she watched in amazement as they tried shaking everything, from cucumbers to peaches to tomatoes.)

But it turns out that this directive about coloring meals is not as hard as it seems at first. The problem most people have is this: When they think of fruits and veggies, they envision only the produce section of their grocery store. While fresh is great, it's not the only way to work in fruits and vegetables.

So we should think outside the produce section. A few of Leslie's ideas: Mix a can of diced tomatoes with some chopped onion as a topping for fish. Slice up fresh veggies and toss them lightly with olive oil, then grill them on foil next to the meat. Eat soup year-round and toss in a serving of beans or ½ cup of frozen vegetables while it heats.

Look out. Now Leslie's on a roll with her fruit and vegetable suggestions. Here are her ideas for every meal:

BREAKFAST

- Add a sliced banana to cereal.
- Add berries to yogurt.
- Have a glass of tomato juice.
- Add salsa to scrambled eggs.
- Top a waffle with sliced peaches (fresh or frozen).

LUNCH

- Put extra veggies on your sandwich, like cucumber or shredded carrots, which are great in pocket bread.
- Use hummus or refried beans as a spread instead of mayo or mustard.
- Have some raw veggies with lunch instead of chips or pretzels.

- Add grapes, melon, or pineapple to your salad.

- Blend frozen fruit with seltzer water for a peppy, colorful beverage.

- Have a pickle. It's a vegetable!

DINNER

- Make room on the grill for vegetables, not just meat.

- Add craisins or golden raisins to a rice pilaf.

- Try mango, peach, or pineapple salsa on chicken or fish.

- Prepare roasted vegetables. Put veggies in a single layer on a cookie sheet, drizzle with 1 tablespoon of olive oil, season with sea salt and pepper, and roast in a 450°F oven for 5 to 7 minutes.

- Add frozen vegetables or beans to spaghetti sauce.

When you add fruits and vegetables to your diet, you usually take something else away. If you make room for extra veggies on your plate, there's less room for the starch. In an ideal world, a higher-calorie food with less nutrients gets subbed out for the colorful stuff. And that's an easy way to whack a few hundred calories off your total intake during a week.

Leslie's Lessons: "Frozen, canned, dried, jarred, prepackaged—those are all fine, too! Many people have good intentions: They buy a whole bunch of fresh produce, then they forget to use it and later find it rotting in the bottom of their fridge. Frozen and canned ingredients take the work out of the equation. Chopping tomatoes, for instance, is a pain in the butt. Who has the time? Most people are not soaking dry beans. Canned are fine!"

FRUIT AND VEGGIE PITFALLS

The downside to buying produce that's not fresh is that you're going to have to pick up the package and do that flip-and-read again. It takes only a few seconds to check the label at the store. But many products that masquerade as healthy are carrying a lot of additional baggage.

For instance, if you're going to buy canned pineapple, avoid buying it packed in calorie-laden syrup. Try one in juice instead. Check that the frozen fruit bars have nothing extra added. (Edy's and Breyer's are good bets.) Go for *canned* sweet potatoes, not candied. And when you buy frozen veggies, avoid the ones in heavy sauce. Birds Eye Green Beans and Spaetzle in Bavarian Style Sauce, which made frequent appearances at the dinner table of my youth, packs 150 calories, 7 grams of fat, and 390 milligrams of sodium into a single serving. That extra fat and sodium can sabotage your healthy intentions.

Your serving habits can mess with your calorie total, too. Many people reflexively fix a bowl of veggies to serve the family and plop half a stick of butter (which would be 400 calories) on top. It's simply not necessary. A skimpy olive oil drizzle in the preparation will save you tons of calories.

While we're on the topic of calories yet again, bear in mind that a small piece of fruit, like a pear, apple, or 5-inch banana, is 60 calories. A serving of vegetables is 25 calories. That is why we advise you to max out at two, possibly three servings of fruit per day when you're watching your weight. But you can go unlimited on the veggies—except for potatoes and corn, which are higher in starchy calories.

RUNNING MAKES ME HUNGRY!

All well and good, you say. But with this running program? I'm hungry all the time!

You're not alone in that. Many people trying to lose weight have experienced exercise making them hungry. A widely discussed and controver-

> The most important thing to remember is that exercise has so many health benefits. Even the people who are skeptical about how much it contributes to weight loss say you should exercise anyway.

sial 2009 *Time* magazine cover story that proclaimed "Why Exercise Won't Make You Thin" was predicated on the notion that all this exercise just makes us famished. The *New York Times Magazine* picked up the thread in an April 2010 piece, "Weighing the Evidence on Exercise," which discussed how increases in exercise can stimulate hormones associated with appetite.

Reading this kind of reporting can make anyone a little discouraged. But don't hang up the running shoes just yet. You can handle this, and you can outwit your hormones.

The most important thing to remember is that exercise has so many health benefits; even the people who are skeptical about how much it contributes to weight loss say you should exercise anyway. As you well know, the effects of exercise on cardiovascular health, bone density, stress levels, and even mental acuity make it an invaluable part of your daily routine. And researchers agree that exercise is crucial for *maintaining* weight loss.

Now, not everyone experiences the increased hunger effect after exercise. Several people on the test panel said their appetites were actually suppressed after running and walking. They were decidedly unenthused by food when they were done running. Lucky them. At the very least they should have a large glass of water to rehydrate after their runs, but otherwise they can enjoy the not-so-hungry feeling for a while.

For the rest of us, we offer this: *RYBO* takes such a gradual approach to building up that we believe the postexercise hunger pangs aren't overwhelming. Between Stages 5 and 6, we added 1 minute of running. Between Stages 6 and 7, there are 3 more minutes of running. That shouldn't greatly alter your body's chemistry from week to week.

Still hungry, you say? Do another couple of days of food logging and look at the calorie distribution throughout the day. Are you eating enough before you exercise? If you're not, you're more likely to be ravenous after exercise. (Chances are, even if you weren't running, you might be starving by that point in the day anyway.) So experiment with the timing and quantity of your eating to see if you can get your postrun hunger pangs under control.

THE POSTWORKOUT SNACK

By filling up the tank again with a satisfying postrun snack, you'll be better able to stave off the munchies that hit later. If you're the type who finds that running makes you hungry, try to eat within 30 minutes of finishing your workout. Aim for a balance of healthy carbohydrates and protein, which will make you feel satisfied. First drink water to give your stomach the feeling of "yes, there's something in there."

Leslie's suggestions for postrun snacks:

- 10-ounce bottle of 1% chocolate milk (170 calories, 10 grams of protein)

- 1 container of strawberry Greek yogurt (140 calories, 14 grams of protein)

- Small skinny latte (90 calories, 8 grams of protein)

Later on, as you become more advanced and are running 5, 6, 7 miles in a workout, the postworkout snack becomes mandatory. You'll need to eat something within 30 minutes of finishing; aim for 35 grams of carbohydrate and 12 to 15 grams of protein. This will top off your muscle glycogen stores and help with protein resynthesis.

At the beginner level, a small postrun snack is a way to troubleshoot, to keep you from overeating later on. It takes the edge off your hunger.

Bottom line: Don't use hunger as an excuse to curtail your exercise. Give it some time, juggle when and how much you eat, and experiment with snacks. You'll find a schedule that works for you.

> Don't use hunger as an excuse to curtail your exercise.

NOEL CAROL, 57

Job: Social worker and supervisor, New Jersey Department of Human Services; mother of three and grandmother of one

Goals: To run 30 minutes straight and finish a 5-K

Starting weight: 184 pounds

Ending weight: 174 pounds

Starting waist: 33¾ inches

Ending waist: 31 inches

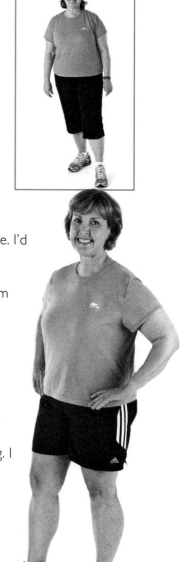

Small Food Changes: I cut back from two glasses of wine to one, and I stopped buying cheese. I'd want to eat it all in one sitting.

Confidence Building: I've stopped feeling like I'm too old or too fat to run. I've gotten over my self-consciousness.

The Great Outdoors: I often feel that my running has taken on a rhythm. I am not thinking about the run but enjoying the moment (even if I am still really slow). My aerobic strength has improved immensely, and my legs feel very strong. I find myself concentrating on the beauty that surrounds me. It is the best time of the day!

Secret Weapon: My blog! I started a blog to write about my running and goals. A few of my friends read it, and they've been inspired to get moving, too. Making my hopes and struggles public keeps me going. My best friend growing up just ran her first continuous mile. I'm so proud of her. (http://grammiegetsalife.blogspot.com)

The Next Goal: I signed up for a marathon in 7 months! I have always wanted to finish a marathon. I don't care how long it takes me; I just want to finish. I have one friend doing it with me and two more who are considering it.

Getting Out There: On the days I really don't want to exercise, I just start slow. If I'm still having a hard time, I'll stop. But I've found that many of my best workouts have been on those days that I didn't feel like it.

Chapter 8

Sometimes It's Not About the Scale

When Colleen, 35, first started running in the spring of 2010, she was enduring rough times. Both her parents had recently passed away, and she was going through a divorce. As a bookkeeper for an accounting firm and a mom of a 6-year-old, she had a lot to juggle, all with an extra burden of sadness shading her days.

Somehow, through all the stress, she had the clarity to sign up for First Strides, the beginning running class. She also enrolled in our test panel. She met with the class for one run a week and did two other weeknight runs by herself at about 9:00 p.m., when it wasn't so hot and she could blow off steam from her packed days.

Running soon became her refuge. "About 5 weeks in, that's when it really hit me," she says. "It was just this great feeling of accomplishment. I was actually doing this." Even her soon-to-be-ex-husband noticed her resolve and expressed his admiration.

Amid the loss, she found something she had gained. "Running is a mood lifter for me," she says now. The sport also completely upended the way Colleen thinks about herself. "I was never the athletic type," she says. "I was always a lazy person, in all honesty. I couldn't even run around the track one time without feeling like I was going to die. But to finally be running and not be out of breath? It just came together."

WHEN IT'S NOT ABOUT THE SCALE

The external transformation wasn't as noticeable. With all that was going on in her personal life, Colleen admitted she couldn't devote too much energy to changing her eating habits. She started the 12-week program at 163 pounds.

And at the end she weighed . . . drumroll, please . . . 163 pounds.

This is what happens in real life. Sometimes you focus on losing weight and you lose weight. Sometimes you focus on doing something healthy for yourself and you lose weight in the process. Or you don't. For Colleen, the number on the scale was an afterthought. Running was the

I Was Terrible at Sports Until I Tried Running

I heard sentiments similar to Colleen's over and over from people on the test panel: "I never played sports as a kid." "In gym class I was picked last for teams." "I was always on the sidelines."

It seems like the more sports-averse you were as a child, when you finally discover you can run, you embrace the sport like a long-lost brother. Amy N. put it this way: "I never did well in sports like basketball. You had to be really aggressive and in people's faces and trying to steal the ball and stuff like that. I don't like a competitive setting. With running, I'm setting my own goals. I'm pushing myself. If I don't hit a goal, I'm not letting anyone else down. If I triumph, then it's just me."

I'm not usually sentimental about running. I love it and I love what it does for me, but I can't say I get misty-eyed when I talk about it. When I hear Colleen and Amy talk about running, however, I'm impressed. It's like they've opened this gift, and inside they've discovered fitness, self-satisfaction, and a whopping sense of accomplishment.

Like I've said before, you can't really get that from an elliptical machine.

point, something to be happy about. It was also a pleasant surprise to Colleen because she had never been active before.

OUTRUNNING YOUR PAST

So many beginning runners, especially those who never did sports before, lack self-assurance when they're starting out. They feel like frauds, like someone is going to unveil them as the couch potatoes they used to be, or that tyrannical gym teacher who tortured them in seventh grade is going to jump out just down the trail.

Sometimes when the running gets easier for beginners, it has nothing to do with their physical condition. They just get more confident. Noel Carol noticed that. Like everyone, she started out running for 1-minute intervals. A few months later, she was routinely running 30 to 45 minutes without stopping to walk. What's the difference? "I think the confidence that I can do it," she says. "And not feeling like I'm too old or too fat or too slow. Midway through, I began to lose my self-consciousness. I didn't care anymore because I was doing something I liked doing."

Beginning runners have to complete a certain number of runs, runs that get ever longer, before they believe they belong. The workouts in this chapter are a big deal because you're knocking on the door of 10 minutes of running. And that's a point when a person starts to admit, "Looks like I'm for real with this running thing!"

STAGE 8 WORKOUT

- Walk for 2 minutes. Run for 9 minutes.

- Repeat that sequence one more time.

- Then walk for 2 minutes, run for 8 minutes.

- End with 3 minutes of walking.

Total workout time: 35 minutes, 26 of which are running.

Do this workout at least three or four times in a week before moving on to the next stage.

By the time you're reading this chapter, you've been at this exercising routine for at least 7 weeks, maybe more if you've taken some extra weeks to get used to a particular workout. Let's see: Seven weeks and you're getting out there for at least three—better yet, four—exercise sessions per

COLLEEN, 36

Job: Bookkeeper and mother of a 6-year-old

Goals: Lose weight, increase my energy and endurance, and improve my overall health and well-being

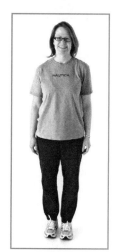

Starting weight: 163

Ending weight: 163

Wow! Moment: I was never athletic at all growing up. Truthfully, I was kind of lazy. So it's been a surprise how great running feels.

Night Moves: I find it easier to run at night after my daughter goes to bed. In the summer, it's cooler in the dark. It's so peaceful and it's a time for me to tune into myself. I do wear a reflective vest to be visible to cars.

Staying Vigilant: I went on vacation during the summer, and while I was away, I did not care about my eating. I was doing so much walking that I figured that I could splurge a bit. It didn't work that way, and I put on weight. I have taken it off again, but I'll know in the future to be more careful.

Food Changes: My diet is a work in progress, but cutting back on my snacking during the day has really helped me. I try to get more fruits and veggies in at every meal.

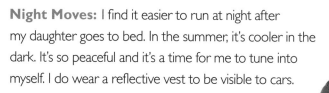

week. That means you've been out there at least 21 to 28 times. You're on a roll.

Really, now, isn't this starting to feel better? If you intend to run but can't make it, don't you sort of miss it? That's what happened to Colleen.

You'll notice that this workout and the next one are very similar. So we're putting them together in the same chapter. Don't get skimpy on us and try to do them both in a week. Take at least a full week with each stage.

LETTING YOUR MIND FLOAT

Here's something else that's happening as the workouts pile up: While you're running, your mind is wandering. You're not so focused on the numbers on the watch anymore. When the running interval is only 3 minutes or less, you can stay hyperfocused on the time. You look at your watch every 30 seconds or so and know exactly how much longer you have until you can walk. It's like a kid on a long car trip: "Dad, are we there yet? Mom, are we there yet?" Is the running part over?

That all changes once the running segments start to tally 7, 8, 9 minutes and longer. You can't be constantly on a countdown.

In fact, a few people on our test panel told us that when they got to this level, they started feeling annoyed by having to look at their watch. So they'd do the walking warmup, then start running—and would often

---

Budd's Buzz: "By the time you run for 8 minutes, you might not be able to see off in the distance how far you're going. And your mind starts to drift. And that's when it's pretty cool. You don't have to concentrate on 'I'm running, I'm running, I'm running' the whole time. You can let yourself daydream, solve a few problems. You don't have to keep looking at your watch because you know that it's going to be a while."

---

unknowingly exceed the prescribed running interval because they weren't so focused on time.

The first time this happens, it's very cool.

So here's the next stage workout. You're getting closer each week to the ultimate prize: a 30-minute nonstop run.

STAGE 9 WORKOUT

- Walk for 1 minute. Run for 9 minutes.
- Repeat that sequence two more times.
- End with 3 minutes of walking.

Total workout time: 33 minutes, 27 of which are running.

Do this workout at least three or four times in a week before moving on to the next stage.

In 9 minutes of running, you're covering a mile if you're speedy, probably closer to 0.7 mile if you're taking a more comfortable pace. Either way, it's a significant amount of ground under your feet. Then you multiply that by three segments and you've gone at least 2, possibly closer to 3, miles.

Now remember what we've said all along. The most important thing is just getting out there at least three—better yet, four—times a week. Consistency is the key. This plan is not set in stone. Your improvement does not have to be a straight line up. You can mix and match old workouts while getting used to the new ones in this chapter.

But there's a fine line between progressing conservatively and being complacent. You're the one who has to figure out where that line is. When Budd works with beginning runners, he has to give them a verbal kick in the pants from time to time, because he knows they are capable of more than they let on.

Consistency is the key.

> **Budd's Buzz:** "Every once in a while, I coach a runner and I need to say, 'You've been at this stage for 3 weeks now; you've got to move up, let's go!' Those are the people who need to get an attitude, a nothing-can-stop-me attitude. Really! Don't give in. Don't settle for less. Set a goal and accomplish it. Your goal is to run for 30 minutes. Let's keep going!"

TAKE GOOD CARE

I have only one concern with Colleen's transformation from self-proclaimed "lazy person" to runner: those after-dark runs. There's no problem with running at night as long as you take some precautions. Make sure you wear reflective clothing, and stick to well-lit areas so you don't fall over a branch or uneven road that you can't see.

All runners need to keep safety in mind. Avoid running during the hottest times of the day, tell someone where you're going and how long you'll be gone, and carry identification with you. *Runner's World* editors love the Road ID, a little metal tag that attaches with Velcro to your shoelaces and informs anyone reading it who you are and whom to call in case, heaven forbid, you can't speak for yourself.

Drivers aren't getting any better. They're the biggest hazard we face. Run on the left side of the road so you're facing traffic, pick routes with wide shoulders, turn down the iPod so you can hear cars coming, and be alert as they pass you. It's a sad state of affairs that we have to worry about drivers distracted by texting, but we do. So keep your wits about you. And keep running.

HOLY COW!

Here's the million-dollar question: How much protein do you need each day?

Leslie's answer: A physically active person (and yes, you qualify if

Muscle It!

For more than a decade, through the Atkins craze and the South Beach Diet, Americans have been viewing carbohydrates with some suspicion. The health-conscious among us have learned that protein—lean protein—is good for us. But even with all the positive press protein has been getting, it's hard to eat enough of it unless we give it some serious thought and planning.

you're already into Chapter 8 of *RYBO*) needs ½ gram for every pound of body weight. So a 200-pound person would need 100 grams of protein; a 160-pounder would need 80.

Now, what if you currently weigh 180 pounds but are hoping to reach 160? Use the goal weight in your calculation and aim for 80 grams.

Does that seem like a ton of protein to you? Because it does to me. And chances are, you're not currently getting what you need.

Why so much? Protein is a versatile, kick-butt nutrient.

- It's an essential building block for a healthy body because it helps build muscle and preserve lean body mass. You need those muscles, remember, so you can run and do everything else you want to do.

- Like fiber, protein takes longer to leave the stomach, which makes you feel fuller longer. And if you feel satisfied for a longer period of time, you're less likely to overeat.

- The body works harder digesting protein, and it's burning a few extra calories during digestion. (It's that thermogenic effect of food again, as we discussed with fiber.) We love that kind of food because it boosts metabolism without our having to do anything. You get more bang for the buck. Carbs, on the other hand, don't make you feel very full, and they pass through your system easily, requiring less work for your digestive system to process them.

"Okay," you might be saying, "so I'm convinced. Those are all good reasons to get more protein." Good. Now here's how you do it.

NOT ALL PROTEIN IS CREATED EQUAL

First, you want to be discriminating about your protein. You want to get the right kind, the kind that isn't accompanied by whopping amounts of fat, sodium, extra calories, and a side of fries. We're talking lean meat, low-fat dairy, whole grains, beans, and nuts, not Burger King or an extra-cheese pizza from Dominos.

> You want to have some protein with every meal.

Second, you want to have some with every meal. And that's where a lot of people have trouble.

But as we know, this whole *RYBO* program is about paying attention and training the brain as well as the gut and the mouth. We can handle this. So let's get to it.

Leslie's Lessons: "A lot of the research on nutrition and weight loss has shown that it's not just the amount of protein that matters but how and when people consume it. The idea is, in order to optimize protein nourishment for your cells, you have to have some as part of every meal. That's a better way of doing it, rather than eating very little protein during the day, then at night sitting down to a cow or a fowl. The downside is it requires a little more attention to detail."

MUSCLE YOUR MEALS

Here, Leslie lists some easy ways to pack more protein punch into your meals and snacks throughout the day.

BRAWNY BREAKFASTS

- Two hard-boiled eggs with a slice of toast
- Two slices of part-skim mozzarella, provolone, or Swiss melted on a whole wheat English muffin
- Smoothie made with 8 ounces of fat-free milk, 6 ounces of yogurt, and ½ cup of frozen fruit, blended together
- Two low-fat beef, turkey, or soy sausage links with a whole wheat waffle
- ½ cup of cottage cheese topped with ¼ cup of granola and ½ cup of sliced fruit

LEAN, MEAN LUNCHES

- Salad topped with a 3-ounce can or packet of tuna, salmon, or chicken
- Wrap with ½ cup of vegetarian refried beans, ½ cup of veggie crumbles, and ¼ cup of shredded light Cheddar cheese with salsa
- Vegetable omelet with 3 eggs, ½ cup of frozen vegetables, and 1 tablespoon of Parmesan cheese
- Sandwich made with ½ cup of shaved ham or smoked turkey with barbecue sauce added (for a different flavor)
- 1 cup of chili made with lean ground meat, ground turkey breast, veggie crumbles, or texturized vegetable protein (TVP); taco seasoning or chili powder; kidney beans; and chopped tomatoes; served with ½ cup of brown rice or over a small baked potato

PROTEIN-PACKED SNACKS

- ½ cup of edamame with sea salt
- ½ cup of cottage cheese seasoned with dried soup mix (try Rachel's Cucumber Dill flavor) and veggies to dip
- Special K or Kashi bar
- Single-serving container of Greek yogurt
- 2 slices of low-fat cheese with an apple

- 1 cup of fat-free milk with ¾ cup of Special K cereal
- Shake made with 1 scoop of whey protein isolate, 1 cup of fat-free chocolate milk, and crushed ice
- 2 tablespoons of peanut butter on a banana
- Turkey or chicken jerky
- ¼ cup of roasted soy nuts

PROTEIN SNACKS ON THE GO

- To-go packets of whey protein isolate mixed into water
- Mini-bag of high-fiber cereal added to yogurt
- Hard-boiled egg
- String cheese

DYNAMITE DINNERS

- 5-ounce piece of chicken or fish, broiled and topped with Cajun seasoning, served with 1 cup of vegetables and a small sweet potato
- Stir-fry with 1 cup of frozen shrimp and 2 cups of vegetables over ⅔ cup of brown rice
- 4-ounce burger (that's cooked weight, so start with 6 ounces raw) on a whole grain bun
- Salad with 4 ounces of sliced steak, ½ cup of black beans, and ½ cup of corn salsa over mixed greens
- 2 chicken-and-vegetable kebabs made with 5 ounces of meat (start with 7 ounces raw) and served over quinoa for even more protein

COUNT PROTEIN FIRST, THEN CALORIES

By adding the right kind of protein to your diet along with plenty of fruits and veggies, your calorie total for the day will naturally fall in line. If you eat enough protein, you're just not as hungry. And trust me when I say

that it's more fun to make sure you're getting *enough* of something than to hold back
from consuming too much. Addition is
great; restriction is annoying.

> If you eat enough protein,
> you're just not as hungry.

So let's see how this might work. Time to put myself on the hot seat
here. My old diet, before Leslie powered up my protein, might have looked
something like this.

TIME	FOOD	AMOUNT	PROTEIN	CALORIES
7:00 a.m.	Multi-Bran Chex	1 serving	3 grams	160
	Fat-free milk	8 ounces	8 grams	90
	Grapefruit	½ fruit	0 grams	20
10:00 a.m.	Low-fat yogurt	1 container	5 grams	130
	Quaker Brown Sugar Oatmeal Squares cereal, dry	½ cup	3 grams	105
1:00 p.m.	Deli turkey	2 ounces	9 grams	60
	Whole wheat bread	2 slices	8 grams	200
	Low-fat mayo	1 tablespoon	0 grams	35
	Lettuce	1 piece	negligible	negligible
	Cucumber	3 slices	negligible	negligible
	Bosc pear	1 medium	0.5 gram	80
4:00 p.m.	Chocolate sandwich cookies	2	1.33 grams	120
7:00 p.m.	Baby carrots	8	0 grams	20
	Pasta	3 ounces	10.5 grams	300
	Vodka sauce	½ cup	2 grams	120
	Kraft Parmesan cheese	2 teaspoons	2 grams	20
	Steamed broccoli	½ cup	2 grams	30
9:00 p.m.	Edy's vanilla light ice cream	1 cup	6 grams	200
	Hershey's chocolate syrup	1 tablespoon	0.5 gram	50
TOTAL			61 grams	1,740

I'm short of the 65 grams of protein I should be getting. I know I'm not alone in this, either. Leslie looked at the food logs of everyone on the test panel, and nearly everyone was struggling to get the protein they needed. Now that Leslie has given my meals a protein makeover, here's what I'm looking at.

TIME	FOOD	AMOUNT	PROTEIN	CALORIES
7:00 a.m.	Oatmeal	½ cup	5 grams	150
	Fat-free milk	1 cup	8 grams	90
	Almonds	14	3 grams	85
	Strawberries/blueberries	½ cup	0.5 gram	50
10:00 a.m.	Plain Greek yogurt	6 oz	14 grams	90
	Honey	2 tsp	0 grams	40
1:00 p.m.	Deli turkey	2 oz	9 grams	60
	Naturally Slender American cheese	1 slice	5 grams	60
	Whole wheat bread	2 slices	8 grams	200
	Hummus	2 Tbsp	2 grams	50
	Lettuce	1 piece	negligible	negligible
	Cucumber	3 slices	negligible	negligible
	Bosc pear	1 medium	0.5 gram	80
	Chocolate sandwich cookie	1 cookie	0.67 gram	60
4:00 p.m.	Kashi almond bar	1 bar	6 grams	140
7:00 p.m.	Baby carrots	8	0 grams	20
	Cottage cheese	2 oz	5.5 grams	45
	Chicken breast	14 oz	26 grams	110
	Israeli couscous	⅓ cup	6 grams	190
	Salad	1 cup	negligible	negligible
	Newman's Own Family Style Italian dressing	2 Tbsp	0 grams	90
9:00 p.m.	Fat-free milk	1 cup	8 grams	90
	Hershey's chocolate syrup	1 Tbsp	0.5 gram	50
TOTAL			108 grams	1,750

This is not a radical makeover. I'm making small swaps at each meal—adding a few nuts, a little low-fat cheese, and lean meat; benching the white pasta; swapping a Greek yogurt for the regular kind, which lowers the calories and ups the protein. Together these changes get me well over the 65 grams I need per day to fuel my exercise and schlep the kids around. And, frankly, I'm less hungry. It's not so hard to go a few hours between meals, and at night I'm not so tempted to explore what's in the freezer. A glass of chocolate milk satisfies my sweet tooth.

Just as happens with fruits and veggies, when you make room for protein, something has to go. Usually it's the carbs, which are higher in calories. Very few people in America have to worry about not getting enough carbohydrate. If you're concerned with that, you're probably an ultramarathoner. For now, if you do it right, swapping in the protein and swapping out the carbs, your total calorie intake will be reduced. And this is what you're after.

THE WEEKEND TRAP

Leslie looks at food logs like a stockbroker watches the Dow. Every week she gets them from her clients in Pittsburgh. With a quick scan of a page, she can get a sense of where the problem areas are for someone who overeats or where an athlete complaining of fatigue is lacking a certain type of nutrient.

With the everyday folks, one pattern pops up over and over again.

The weekdays are healthy. The weekends are pretty ugly.

In some ways, that's completely understandable. Our weekdays are so tightly structured that there's not a lot of time for deviating from the plan. If you have only 15 minutes for breakfast at home and then it's off for a busy day, you're going to eat whatever healthy choices you've stocked for yourself.

But on weekends, we have a little more time and flexibility. We have

FOOD TALK Drink It!

Protein is not the only thing you need a lot of. You need plenty of liquid—the right kind of liquid.

Ninety ounces per day for women. For men, 125 ounces.

Gulp.

Why so much? In a nutshell, you need liquid so your body works the way it's supposed to work. Those 90 ounces are the Institute of Medicine's recommendation on what a person needs each day for cellular functioning, to aid digestion, to maintain appropriate core body temperature, and for proper joint lubrication. You need to be hydrated to exercise, too. So for all these reasons, the body needs a lot of the wet stuff throughout the day.

Now here's the good news: Everything except alcohol counts.

Those 90 or 125 ounces don't have to be water alone. Coffee counts. Milk counts. The juice in a juicy pear and the liquid in your soup count. So you're probably not as far from the total as you might have thought initially.

The point is this: Have a big glass of water with every meal. Not only will it help with all your body's functions, but it will contribute to satiety, which is that feeling of fullness. "It's a relatively transient sensation, to feel fuller when drinking water," Leslie says, "but water takes up more room in the stomach than a bowl of potato chips does."

Cheers!

special occasions galore: weddings and baby showers, birthday parties, graduations. There's coffee hour after church—and I've never seen much besides Danish and doughnuts at a coffee hour. Or there's the family ritual of going to a diner on a weekend morning or eating buttered popcorn at the movies.

> You need liquid so your body works the way it's supposed to work.

Weekends are full of challenges to navigate.

Harrison, one of the test panelists and a law student, was incredibly disciplined throughout the week. He logged his food intake down to a single Gummi Bear he'd eat before class—no joke. He knew that the cooked weight of his pork chop was 4½ ounces.

But come Saturday he'd eat a large Italian hoagie from a sub shop. Dinner was at a Mexican restaurant, where he'd dive into three chicken-and-cheese burritos with sauce, refried beans, and a 12-ounce margarita, enjoying the chips and salsa at the table.

Leslie's advice for Harrison might seem unconventional, but here it is: He should have the Mexican on Wednesday. If he can, hold himself to just two burritos.

Then, when the weekend comes, he won't feel like he has been deprived all week and he can even out his calorie intake.

On the next page, Leslie offers her rationale for managing weekends.

Leslie's Lessons: "I would rather someone eat the same amount of food every day than be good during the week and very bad on the weekend. We need to bargain. So if cake or other goodies are not around during the week and they are on the weekend, then you decide which item or items you cannot live without. For instance, have the slice of birthday cake, but then have the burger without the bun and eat a salad with it. Or go for the two glasses of champagne, but then have chicken, fish, or meat with vegetables, salad, and fruit, and forgo the bread, rice, pasta, and potatoes.

"If your normal Saturday routine is to start with the Belgian waffle and it goes downhill from there, maybe try having your weekday yogurt with bran on a Saturday morning. Even if you have a meal later that's a little more indulgent, it hasn't been a day that's 100 percent indulgent.

"Allow yourself a little flexibility during the week, too. If you have a treat on Thursday, like that Belgian waffle, then you won't feel so deprived when the weekend comes and feel like you deserve to overeat. Find a middle ground. Get out of this black-and-white and good-and-bad mind-set. I'd prefer to see the calories even out from weekday to weekend rather than this roller-coaster."

SECRETS OF THE TEST PANEL

HARRISON, 24

Job: Law student

Goals: To lose weight and increase my stamina

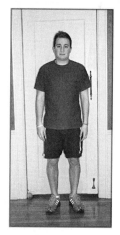

Starting weight: 165 pounds

Ending weight: 155 pounds

Back in the Day: I had gotten up to 200 pounds in January 2010. I lost 35 pounds just by watching what I ate, but then I plateaued. Running helped me take off the last 10 pounds.

Becoming a Runner: I had tried running a few times before, but I would just go out and run, with no plan and no direction. That didn't work for me. I needed a training schedule to follow. It's easier to accomplish a goal that way.

Secret Weapon: Chopsticks. I'm not very good at using them, so they force me to eat slowly.

Beware the Weekends: Weekends can be tough because it's really easy to go out with friends for lunch and dinner. I learned from Leslie to try to stay a little more consistent, so the healthy eating carries over from weekday to weekend.

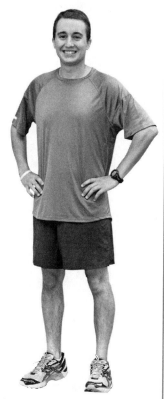

Photo: Nick Galac

Chapter 9

Boredom Busters

This training program doesn't give a hoot about distance, as you've no doubt noticed by now. We only measure in time—how many minutes you can run. The next time your smart-aleck brother-in-law questions how far you're running? Tell him you don't know and you don't care.

There are only three times when distance matters. The first is in your rough calculations of how many calories you're burning. Gotta have an approximate distance to do that math. The second time is for races. Some-day soon you'll run your first 5-K, not your first 30-minute race.

And the third time distance matters is when you run over a limited route. The more you do it, the more likely you are to get tired of that par-ticular geography. The reality is you're probably running at least 2 miles with every workout. It might be closer to 3, depending on your speed. Add in the walking portions and you're definitely covering some ground.

If you're running around a quarter-mile track, you probably weren't bored back in the beginning when you were going around six times per workout. But now that you're approaching 12 laps per workout, you might be feeling a little antsy. Same thing goes if you're running a 1-mile fitness trail over and over. By the 12th time you've done it in a week, you are probably wondering what's out there, over that horizon.

Some people can run the same route at the same time of day week after week, month after month, and never feel the slightest bit of tedium or urge to skip a workout. Good for them. (These are the same people, by the way, who are completely internally motivated and never crave an ice cream sandwich.)

Most of us feel stale a little more easily than that. Here are a few ways to change up your running if you need a kick in the pants:

Explore a new locale. Try the park across town, test out a trail you've never been on, or stop in at a runner's shop and ask for some suggestions. Print a course map from a 5-K and experiment with parts of the route. Go to mapmyrun.com and play around with it. See if you can find various routes from your front door that give you between 2 and 3 miles.

Run at a different time of day, if possible. Your familiar route will be cast in a whole new light, literally. Invite different friends to join you.

Lose the watch and try a playlist instead. One test panelist got sick of always looking at her watch, so she programmed different playlists into her iPod instead. The combined duration of the songs totaled the amount of minutes she was supposed to run. Unfortunately, she could find only one song that was exactly 1 minute for the minute-long walking breaks: "Twister" by "Weird Al" Yankovic. "It's a terrible song, really annoying," she says, "but it's the only one I have. You don't want to run to it anyway."

STAGE 10 WORKOUT

- Walk for 2 minutes. Run for 13 minutes.

- Repeat that sequence one more time.

- End with 3 minutes of walking.

Total workout time: 33 minutes, 26 of which are running.

Do this workout at least three or four times in a week
before moving on to the next stage.

I can almost see your brow furrowing as you read the workout. You're reading it twice to make sure your eyes aren't playing tricks on you.

Going from 9 minutes of running in Stage 9 to 13 minutes this week seems like a big step, right? Until now, the biggest change in running between stages has been an additional 2 minutes, so it's understandable if going up 4 minutes in one fell swoop seems like a bit of a shock. But this is not a misprint.

In reality, if you've been pacing yourself and keeping your breathing

Treasure the Compliments

Nothing gets you out the door again faster than if someone notices you're working hard and losing weight. So listen up and take the admiration with a smile and a "thanks." Here's a sampling of the comments our test panelists heard:

> *"I went to a funeral, and my little black dress was a little big. A good friend of mine said, 'You look awesome. I mean, really fabulous.'"*

> *"Without my asking, my running buddy said, 'I can see it in your thighs. You look firmer.'*
> *"I said to her, 'Are you sure?'*
> *"She said, 'Yeah, I can definitely tell.'"*

> *"I went to the pool and a neighbor told me, 'My husband saw you here last week, and he said you look great!'"*

> *"I heard from a coworker that I look svelte. I didn't think people used that word anymore!"*

> *"I have a good friend in Chile, and we Skype regularly. She tells me she can see in my face that I've lost weight."*

With words like these in your head, you'll be just as eager to get out the door as you were back at the beginning. And take the time to compliment yourself. Where's your weight now? Noticing any new muscles that you haven't seen in a few decades? How are you doing on your goals? Can you check any of them off yet?

under control so you're able to talk through the running segments, you should have found a pace that you can maintain for a long time. So the 4-minute leap is more of a mental challenge than a physical one. Maybe you realized a couple of weeks ago that you could probably run longer. But following the plan to the letter, you quit running after 7, then 8, then 9 minutes.

Here's your chance to stretch it out.

The next workout reduces the recovery and tweaks up the running time.

STAGE 11 WORKOUT

- Walk for 2 minutes. Run for 14 minutes.

- Then walk for 1 minute. Run for 14 minutes.

- End with 3 minutes of walking.

Total workout time: 34 minutes, 28 of which are running.

Do this workout at least three or four times in a week
before moving on to the final stage.

Yes, there's 1 measly minute breaking up two 14-minute segments of running. What does this minute do for you? It gives you a mental break. But 60 seconds of walking doesn't give you a whole lot of recovery time when it's sandwiched between all that running.

Some of the people on our test panel loved that minute of walking, *craved* that minute of walking. Others began to see it as a nuisance. Like Becky, who said, "Frankly, I find it takes more effort to get started again after a 1-minute walk than to just keep on going!"

While you're making steady progress on your running, your diet should be rounding into form, too.

FOOD TALK Swap It!

Nine chapters in and you've done a lot of work on your eating. You've calculated your calorie needs, logged your food intake, and planned your shopping. You've examined when you eat, where you eat, and how fast you eat.

All this is an effort to trim a couple of hundred calories per day from your intake. Painlessly, we hope. Even better, maybe your changes are actually tasting good and making you feel better.

There's likely still room for improvement, however, in the "what you eat" category.

FIBER UP!

By now Leslie has taught us the importance of colorful food and high-protein food. Still, there are other occasions when you can make swaps for the better. Get rid of a not-so-healthy something that's part of your daily intake and substitute a healthier, lower-calorie selection.

Dietary fiber is a biggie. Check your bread. Try swapping your stripped-down sandwich bread or toast for something with a little more oomph, which will keep you filled up longer. Aim for 5 grams of fiber per slice.

Cereal, too, might be a place where you can get more bang for your buck. Kellogg's Raisin Bran has 7 grams of fiber and 5 grams of protein per serving. Kellogg's Crispix has only ½ gram of fiber and 2 grams of protein. With breads and cereals, it's well worth spending a few extra seconds at the store to do the flip-and-read and see what you're getting.

An ounce of almonds (about 24) gives you almost 3.5 grams of fiber and 6 grams of protein. The same ounce of potato chips gives you 1 gram of fiber and only 2 grams of protein. They have the same amount of calories, but the almonds stick around your stomach longer. Have the chips and you'll soon be hungry again.

FAT AND FLAVOR

You should be able to shed a few grams of fat without noticing, and you'll cut a bunch of calories. Now, fat is part of what makes food satisfying, so you can't completely rid your diet of it. You need some fat in your food for the aroma, for the feeling in your mouth, to fill you up and make you satisfied. Fat makes food yummy. Any diet that completely strips away the fat won't be sustainable over the long haul.

We went through the fat-free craze back in the late '80s and early '90s, and I still shudder thinking of my mom's pantry populated with Snack-wells, those fat-free cookies that tasted like plasterboard. They had nearly the same number of calories as regular cookies, probably because they had extra sugar to compensate for the missing fat, so they didn't help at all with the deficit we need for weight loss. Same goes for reduced-fat peanut butter. It has the same number of calories per serving as regular peanut butter, so in the fundamental weight-loss equation (calories going in the mouth must be less than calories the body uses), there's no savings with the low-fat version.

How much fat is good for you? We're already asking you to watch your calories and your protein, so you don't have to go crazy counting fat. But you can easily go lower in fat with dairy and meats without missing it. If

> You need some fat in your food for the aroma, for the feeling in your mouth, to fill you up and make you satisfied.

you're on 2% milk and you switch to fat-free, in one serving you'll go from 122 calories to 80 and from 5 grams of fat to zero.

CHECK THE CHEESE

Cheese was a sticking point for several folks on our test panel. Jenn, a 27-year-old scientist, had no idea how much was in a serving size. She could routinely tuck into a block of Cheddar—cut a little slice here, a little slice there. Next thing she knew, half the block was gone in one snack. When she learned what a serving was and held herself to it, she saved a bunch of calories, which went a long way toward explaining her 22-pound weight loss over 12 weeks.

For Roxy, one of the problems was a mountain of cream cheese on her morning bagel. It had been low-fat cream cheese, so she figured it didn't matter how much of it she ate. Leslie convinced her to trade it in for one slice of low-fat mozzarella or Colby melted on her bagel instead. With this swap, Roxy saves about 100 calories.

Noel Carol's solution for the time being is to look the other way as she passes the cheese case in the store. "Swiss is my absolute favorite,"

Leslie's Lessons: "Check out your cheeses and try a light one. Fat-free cheese is beyond hideous. Look for one that, instead of being 100 calories and 9 grams of fat per slice, is 60 calories and 4 grams of fat per slice. There are some light Goudas that are wonderful, some light Swisses are very good, and mozzarella and provolone tend to be part-skim. Cabot Creamery has a Cheddar that's 50% reduced fat, and it doesn't taste like an eraser. Some of the Laughing Cow lights are also tasty. Be sure to check the serving size. If it's a block of cheese, score the bar according to the serving size."

she says ruefully. "But it was very hard for me to eat what is considered a serving. I'd say, 'Oh, I can have another.' So I had to stop buying those things that were hard for me to get control over. Eventually, I hope I can bring them back."

KEEP AN EYE ON THE MEAT

Same rules apply to meat: If you're buying ground beef that's 80% lean, there's a little bad news that comes with that. It's still 20% fat! Try to get meat that's as lean as possible, especially if it's going into a taco or spaghetti sauce. If you're making a burger, you need some fat to keep it from falling apart on the grill. But sub in a little ground turkey with the ground beef and see if anyone in your family even notices. Check out the steaks when you buy them. Are they heavily marbled with white streaks? Can you find a cut that looks leaner, like flank steak or a skirt steak?

Leslie's Lessons: "Many red meats are very lean. You can do a pork loin or an eye round roast, or even a flank steak with a little bit of a vinegar marinade. It's very lean, very low fat, and it's a different look on the plate. It gives you a richer taste than chicken all the time."

Poultry should be skinless, or you can take the skin off before you cook it. The majority of the fat is in the skin. Fish is fine, but only if it's not breaded.

So here's your guideline: Go lower fat on the meat and dairy. You can do so without sacrificing taste. You might have to taste-test

> Go lower fat on the meat and dairy.

a variety of low-fat cheeses—and you might find you stick with the original versions. With items that are high in fat to start with, such as oil, peanut butter, nuts, salad dressing, and snacks, stick with full-fat versions, but carefully monitor serving sizes to keep both calories and fat in check.

REPLICATE THE PACKAGED VERSION

You can reduce a lot of calories just by making something yourself. You know those little envelopes of oatmeal that come in flavors like maple and brown sugar? Try this: Make it yourself with plain oatmeal, add a little bit of sweetener to taste, and do the math on the calories you save. Same goes with yogurt. Rather than buying one with fruit mixed in, which ratchets up the calories, buy plain. Leslie swears by her mix of 1 cup of plain yogurt with ¼ teaspoon of lemon juice, a dash of vanilla extract, and 1 teaspoon of honey.

 FOOD TALK Season It!

If you really wanted, you could come up with a list of foods you like for breakfast, as well as for lunch and a bunch of dinners, then count the calories in each, and mix and match until you get to the total you need for a day. That's not a terrible strategy, especially at first, as you're attempting to get your eating under control and start yourself down the road to losing weight.

But know this: Our mouths get bored. Easily. Our taste buds have ADD. They crave stimulation.

If you don't have enough variety in your diet, sooner or later the boredom is going to get to you. When people go into "diet mode" and all they eat is grilled chicken salad day in and day out, pretty soon the eyes and tongue and brain and gut start begging for something else. It may be salty (like a bag of chips) or sweet and creamy (like ice cream).

Leslie's Lessons: "There's a very fine line between variety and a smorgasbord. When people have too many things around to pick from, then it's really hard to know where to draw the line, and that makes it hard to lose weight. On the other hand, it's a problem to be so limited in your circle of food. The boredom factor creeps in pretty darn quickly, and then you're off and running and looking for other things."

SPICE IT UP

One way to give the same-old, same-old a fresh taste is with spices, a calorie-free strategy for adding pizzazz to your cooking. They couldn't be easier. All you have to do is sprinkle them. You probably mastered that technique as a preschooler in the sandbox.

No need to rush out and buy a bunch of different spices. Start with two or three that you like, or choose a couple of blends. They can be a little pricey, and the shelf life is typically a year. (Mark the date you bought it on the jar so you'll know.) If you eat spices older than a year, they won't make you sick, but the flavors lose their intensity, so there's not much point.

Below, find Leslie's suggestions for using spices and honoring your taste buds.

BREAKFAST

- Add cinnamon to oatmeal or cold cereal.
- Sprinkle hot sauce on eggs to give them a kick.
- Mix vanilla and a splash of lemon juice to plain yogurt, then top with honey and berries.
- Add a dash of ginger to tea.

- Add a little dill to cottage cheese.

- Sprinkle lemon-pepper seasoning on tuna.

- Add a dash or two of Italian seasoning to vegetable soup.

- Try Salad Supreme seasoning on your lettuce, and then just add a little vinegar and olive oil.

- Add fresh herbs such as basil, parsley, or oregano to salads.

- Sprinkle paprika on hummus.

- Add cinnamon to popcorn. For a spicy twist, add chili powder or a little Italian seasoning and Parmesan cheese.

- Stir Mediterranean seasonings into plain yogurt to make a dip for vegetables.

- Add a little ginger, allspice, or cinnamon to a smoothie or hot cocoa.

- Spice up shrimp or fish with Cajun seasoning.

- Pep up grilled chicken with garlic, lemon, olive oil, and Italian seasoning.

- Season vegetables with crushed red-pepper flakes, or roast with cracked pepper, Italian seasoning, and a little sea salt.

- Use curry to flavor rice. Try ½ teaspoon of curry to 2 cups of hot cooked rice.

- Sprinkle Caribbean jerk seasoning on chicken or fish.

GET OUT OF A FOOD RUT

Spices aren't the only way to shock your mouth into happiness. If you feel like your food routine is getting stale, you can give it a jolt—without adding calories, of course.

Leslie's Lessons: "Let's say you're always doing the turkey sandwich for lunch. That's not such a terrible thing, but after a period of time, it really does get tedious. Maybe try a different flavor of turkey breast, such as Cajun or Buffalo roasted. Varying the meat like that doesn't change the calories, it just changes the taste somewhat. Change the bread that you put it on, put a little bit of coleslaw on your sandwich, replace the mayo with a bit of olive tapenade. All of a sudden it takes on a whole new taste, and you're not always staring at that wilted piece of lettuce that looks so incredibly uninspiring, and you're bored before you even eat it."

Diets that rely too much on one ingredient (like cabbage soup) or completely exclude a certain category of nutrients (like fat or carbs) are destined to fail because the mouth wants variety. Or it wants the one thing it's not getting.

Budd and Leslie have tried to make this clear throughout *RYBO*: You want eating—and exercise—habits that are sustainable for months and years, not just a few days.

> You want eating—and exercise—habits that are sustainable for months and years, not just a few days.

Other strategies to vary your eating habits? Change the times. Have lunch for breakfast. Have dinner for lunch. And have breakfast for dinner. Or take your weekend meal and try it midweek. Pancakes on Tuesday? Why not?

Change the look. Try a different bowl or plate. Bring out the fine china. Light some candles. Knock yourself out. It might sound ridiculous, but experiment with anything to keep from getting in a rut.

A WORD ON HUNGER

So, Leslie, what's the deal? Hit me with it straight. Is it possible to lose weight without being hungry? How much sacrifice do we have to make, and how uncomfortable do we have to feel, to shed the pounds?

Like anything, Leslie tells me, it depends on the person. It depends on what habits we had going into this and how much we have to change. Plus everyone has a different perception of hunger.

Here's some good news, however: People who are trying to shed pounds don't want to let themselves get extremely hungry, because then they run the risk of overcompensating and overdoing it when they encounter food again. Best to eat when the hunger-o-meter is at a tolerable 3 or 4 rather than when it's way down at 1 or 2.

Hunger Meter

I is starving—10 is stuffed. Eat when you are at a tolerable 3 or 4 rather than waiting until you are starving (at a 1 or 2). Stop before you reach a 9 or 10.

But the converse applies, too: You don't want to eat so you're absolutely stuffed. Try eating until you're a comfortable 7 or 8, not a jam-packed, can't-possibly-fit-another-bite 9 or 10.

Now, this is where the grazing concept came from. Eat a bunch of little meals so you're never too hungry or too full. Except, as Leslie

> People who are trying to shed pounds don't want to let themselves get extremely hungry.

explained in Chapter 3, if we're always eating, we never learn what hunger feels like, and our minds are completely out of the equation. In addition to potential problems like tooth decay and overstimulation of the gut, any self-awareness about hunger goes completely out the window.

The point of these food lessons is to train your brain to rule your stomach. You might be slightly to moderately hungry at times, but then you know how to feed yourself in a healthy and reasonable way.

25 PERCENT LESS

If you're dutifully counting calories and measuring serving sizes, you know how much food you can eat to lose weight. But if you have a problem with portion control or if you're sick of measuring and counting, you can try the "one-quarter less" rule from Leslie.

When you serve yourself, take out one-quarter of the meal. In other words, put on the plate only 75 percent of what you're used to eating.

Yes, when you cut it down, you'll feel a little hungrier but not uncomfortably so.

It's really just a few less bites per meal. And it's easier to hold some back when you're serving yourself than it is to leave some on your plate. That *really* requires a lot of willpower.

Leslie's Lessons: "I don't think people should be too hungry because, if they are, they aren't going to stick with the program. But I think if people leave every meal feeling absolutely stuffed, then they're eating more than they need. The stomach is like a balloon, and if one repeatedly feeds it to the point of being full, that's what it expects. It anticipates that that's the feeling it's going to have. But if we start to train the gut to get used to having a little less, then the body will adjust to that, too. There have to be sacrifices, but you don't have to starve yourself."

⋯⋯▶ Sensible Snacking

Should hunger pangs hit, stow a few of these snacks in your gym bag or glove compartment or in the fridge at work.

NONPERISHABLE

- 1-ounce packages of ...

    Almonds (164 calories, 6 grams of protein)

    Dry-roasted peanuts (166 calories, 7 grams of protein)

    Pistachios (158 calories, 6 grams of protein)

    Mixed nuts (170 calories, 6 grams of protein)

- Individual bags of popcorn (100 calories, 3 grams of protein)

- SoyJoy bars (130 calories, 4 grams of protein)

- Small boxes of dried fruit such as Sun Maid Raisins (90 calories, 1 gram of protein per 1.5-ounce box)

- Just Tomatoes brand dried vegetables (peas have 100 calories, 7 grams of protein in 1 ounce)

Back to the original question: Do you have to feel hungry to lose weight?

Maybe a little bit, as you train your gut to get used to less food. But you don't have to feel deprived. Like any of the other suggestions in *RYBO,* eating less in a sitting can be a gradual evolution. We don't expect you to dramatically reduce the amount of food in a meal from one day to the next. A little less here, a little less there. Take it slow. Small steps every day.

- 1 ounce of roasted soy nuts (150 calories, 13 grams of protein)
- 1 ounce of dried edamame (124 calories, 11 grams of protein)

PERISHABLE

- 5.3-ounce container of Greek yogurt (86 calories, 14.5 grams of protein)
- Laughing Cow original Swiss cheese wedges (50 calories, 2 grams of protein)
- Laughing Cow Mini Babybel cheese (70 calories, 5 grams of protein)
- 2 tablespoons of hummus (50 calories, 1 gram of protein)
- Dreyer's Fruit Bars (80 calories, no protein)
- 4 ounces of low-fat cottage cheese (80 calories, 11 grams of protein)
- Dill pickles (5 calories, no protein)
- 3 ounces of celery sticks (10 calories, 1 gram of protein)
- 3 ounces of baby carrots (40 calories, 1 gram of protein)
- 12 grape tomatoes (25 calories, no protein)

Leslie's Lessons: "I don't think deprivation is just about the quantity of food consumed; it's also about the choices. The choices that most people make when they're 'dieting' do feel like deprivation because they're limiting what they're eating, not just in volume, but in the types of food. If it's just a salad all the time or a piece of chicken all the time, that's deprivation. If you say, 'I really want that piece of cake, but I'm willing to have less of it,' you won't feel so deprived."

DONNA, 50

Job: Administrative assistant at a ski area

Goals: Increase my speed and run a marathon someday

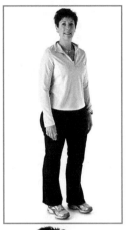

Starting weight: 172 pounds

Ending weight: 158 pounds

Starting waist: 31 inches

Ending waist: 29 inches

Biggest Challenge: Running alone. I work all day in an office by myself, so when I get home, I don't like to run alone. But I don't know anyone near me who runs. My husband will join me sometimes, and I joined a beginning running class, but I have to drive a long way to get there.

What Worked: Increasing my protein intake in the morning. I know you're not supposed to eat in the car, but I have a long commute, so I'll eat a protein bar with a glass of skim milk while driving, and it fills me up for hours.

Words to Live By: "Take care of your body. It's the only place you have to live." —Jim Rohn

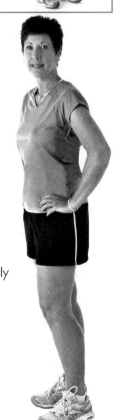

Sweat Strategy: I bought very small microfiber hand towels, and I'll tuck one in my waistband. They are extremely lightweight, and I use them to wipe the sweat while I'm running. I got them at the dollar store.

Dealing with Hills: Some of the hills in my neighborhood are brutal. For a while, I was driving someplace flat for my run. Now I'll attempt the hills. I'll pick a tree off in the distance, and I'll tell myself, "Just get to that point and then you can stop and walk." But sometimes I don't need to stop. I'll get there and find I can keep going. I did a 5-mile race this year, and there were some hills toward the end of the course. The ladies around me were struggling with them, but I found I had no problem.

Tunes for the Tough Times: I love Melissa Etheridge's song "I Run for Life." I'll always program that to play near the end of my run. It gives me incentive to finish strong.

Chapter 10

"The more I run, the more I want to run, and the more I live a life conditioned and influenced and fashioned by my running. And the more I run, the more certain I am that I am heading for my real goal: to become the person I am." —George Sheehan, MD, beloved former *Runner's World* columnist

Don't Stop Now

I made plans with some members of the test panel to do a 5-K race one evening in July. It was a low-key, no-frills affair, part of a series of 5-K races the Lehigh Valley Road Runners hosts Wednesday evenings in the summer. Entrants get a chance to try to run a little faster while enjoying the camaraderie of other runners.

Then a heat wave hit.

It was epic. Temperatures reached 100 degrees, humidity was high, and stepping outside of the air-conditioning seemed like putting a ski mask over your face. Weather forecasters warned everyone to stay inside because the air quality was only slightly better than a smoky bar. So I e-mailed everyone on the test panel and let them off the hook. "No problem if you don't feel like running," I wrote, hoping they'd all bag it. I sure as heck didn't want to go.

A few opted out, but four of them stuck with it, even when the race committee decided to hold the event as a fun run, without entry fees, numbers, or scoring. Their friends and spouses warned them they were crazy. "Ah, if we have to, we'll walk," Becky told me. "At least the sun shouldn't be so bad at that time of day." Talk about looking on the bright side. "When did these test panel volunteers get so darn optimistic anyway?" I grumbled to myself.

There we were, the five of us plus a few friends, wearing shades and baseball hats, carrying our own water, jogging and walking along the trail. It was quite a pack, let me tell you. Chatting about work and families and the next races we were planning to run, no one even mentioned that the heat was bothering them.

Dorene even managed to cut 1½ minutes off her time from a 5-K she had run a few weeks earlier, which had been her first ever. Some of these test panelists, I've learned, harbor long-dormant competitive streaks.

No doubt about it: By the end of the program, they were hooked. When you start to identify yourself as a runner, you don't want to miss a chance.

A FINISH LINE AND A STARTING LINE

When you master this week's workout, you're a runner. No matter what anyone else might think, you are.

So this is it. The big one.

Of course, we hope it's not really a finale. We hope this is just the beginning of your life as a runner. Think of all the races you can train for and places you can explore on two feet. Think of all the calories you can still burn.

This is a habit for life. For weight loss maintenance, exercise is a must-do. Of the 5,000 members of the National Weight Control Registry, a group of people who have lost at least 30 pounds and kept the weight off for at least 1 year, 90 percent say they exercise regularly. On average, they exercise an *hour* a day.

> We hope this is just the beginning of your life as a runner.

Remember, we like running because it torches calories like nothing else. You can get a lot done in less time. But there's no rest for the weary.

So as you get ready for your final stage, here's hoping you'll think of this as the beginning, not the end.

STAGE 12 WORKOUT

- Walk for 3 minutes (or until you're good and ready).

- Run for 30 minutes.

- End with 3 minutes of walking.

Total workout time: 36 minutes, 30 of which are running.

Repeat this sequence throughout your whole life.

Budd's Buzz: "For beginners going from 14 minutes to 30 minutes, it's all mental. One hundred percent mental. I hear it all the time. They'll say, 'I've only been running 13, 14 minutes—how can I run all the way to 30?' I explain to them that the 1-minute break they've been taking is like nothing. A 2-minute break is nothing.

"If they're not convinced, I tell them this: 'If you get to 19 minutes and you want to stop for a minute, go ahead.' But no one ever stops. You watch them and they get this look on their faces like 'I'm going to do this.' They are determined. They all have attitudes—if not to start with, then by the end."

When Julie first saw this workout coming on the heels of the Stage 9 workout, she thought I had made a mistake. "There has to be something in between, right?" she asked. "It can't go from 14 minutes of running to 30 minutes of running without a break."

Well, like we mentioned before, in the previous workout you're doing 28 minutes of running. This week it's 30. That's not much of a difference. That 1-minute walk is more a brain breather than a lungs-and-legs break. You don't get a whole lot of rest in 60 seconds.

THE FINAL MATH

Let's take one more look at the calorie burn, this time for 30 minutes of running.

Remember, we've got our 195-pound person, who now weighs 190, and our 155-pound person, who is now 150. I'll still be conservative in the distance covered. At 14 minutes per mile, which is about what our test panelists ran during that heat wave 5-K, you'd cover 2.1 miles in 30 minutes. Add in another 6 minutes of walking at 18-minute pace and you'd cover $1/3$ mile. So here comes the math:

The equation for calories burned while running, you'll remember, is body weight multiplied by 0.75 multiplied by the distance.

So 190 pounds × 0.75 × 2.1 = 299 calories. Add in 33 calories for the walking portion and it's a 332-calorie workout. The 150-pound person burns 236 calories running and 26 walking, which means he or she has blasted 262 calories during that session.

That's pretty darn impressive for a 36-minute workout.

I have to pound this home: The calorie burn here is an approximation. You'd need to know exactly how far you're going to make this math work. But it gives you a ballpark figure. You can see how compared to the 180 and 144 calories burned in Chapter 2 and even the 300 and 240 calories burned in Chapter 6, the total now is way up there. Multiply by four workouts a week and the 190-pound person is kissing 1,325 calories goodbye; that's 1,048 calories for the 150-pounder. Assuming your calorie intake doesn't go up, this strategy will keep the scale moving downward.

As you get faster and cover more distance, you can reap even more rewards from this short workout.

RACE READY

If you didn't feel prepared before, by now you're qualified to attempt a 5-K. It's normal to feel some jitters when you do your first race. Remember these quick pointers on getting to your first finish line:

- Don't try anything unusual for breakfast the morning of the race. Stick to your old routine. You know what works. Ditto for avoiding new shoes, new shorts, new shirts. Go for the tried-and-true.

- Line up about three-quarters of the way back in the pack, so you're behind the speedy guys in singlets and don't get mowed over. But get ahead of the people who are walking the entire way. You can usually tell by the footwear who's been training and who's out for a onetime walk.

- Start out conservatively, even a little slower than your training pace. The goal is to finish your first race happy and upright, and you won't be either of those things if you start out so fast that you've used up all your energy in the first mile. Ignore the pack and set your own pace. After the first mile, if you want to step it up just a wee bit, that's fine. You can speed up slightly again at the 2-mile mark if you feel like you're bursting with energy.

- Put a smile on your face as you cross the finish line. You've just done something incredible, so look the part!

YOUR RUNNING FUTURE

In the coming weeks, we hope that 30 minutes of running will become easy for you. But it might take a while to get there. So going forward, try to organize your week around the principle of "going long" 1 day. Most people have more time for that on the weekend, both for the workout and for a little extra chilling out afterward.

More-experienced runners adapt a weekday run that's fairly routine, then push a little longer on the weekends. For instance, I run 4 easy miles on Monday and Friday, Wednesday I run 5 miles with the middle 3 at a faster clip, and either Saturday or Sunday I try for about 8 slow miles.

How would that look for you? Well, find a weekday workout you can live with. Maybe it's the 2 walk/8 run for 30 minutes. Then perhaps your weekend run is the 30 minutes nonstop. In time, 30 minutes nonstop will feel routine and can become your weekday run.

When test panelist Tammy finished her running class, she settled on 1 minute walking, 10 minutes running as a workout she can finish comfortably. She does that three times a week, then once on the weekend she'll run straight through and push the distance. She has her eyes on a half-marathon.

Find a level where you're comfortable, so you want to keep getting out there. Amy W. settled on 2 minutes of walking, 6 of running for her weekday runs to convince herself to get out of bed in the morning. (It's a mental game. Once she's out there, she finds she can run 10-minute segments.) Try to push yourself week by week, little by little. Don't settle into a comfortable groove for the long haul.

THE NEXT STEPS: RESOURCES FOR THE REST OF YOUR RUNNING LIFE

Running for 30 minutes straight? Check that off. You've done it, and now you're planning your next race. Maybe it's a faster 5-K you're after, or perhaps a local 5-miler or 10-K has piqued your interest. How do you keep improving? Here are the basics for preparing for longer and faster races:

THE LONG RUN

The critical component for success at longer events is building your endurance, and you can do that with runs that gradually get longer. Here's how you build up: Pick 1 day per week and plan to add 5 minutes to that run *every other week* until you reach 1 hour. For instance, if your regular run is 30 minutes, on "long run day," you'll go 35 minutes. Two weeks later, you'll go for 40 minutes. Two weeks after that, you'll go for 45, until you get to 60. On the off weeks—the weeks in between—stick to your regular 30-minute runs.

A little advice: Take it slow. Race distances like 5-milers and 10-Ks are great new distances to tackle. But there's no rush to sign up for a half-marathon or marathon within the first 12 months of your running career. Those challenges can wait—they'll always be there. We've seen plenty of runners get hurt trying to do too much too soon. With patience, you've successfully converted yourself into a runner. Continue to take it slow. Your legs need plenty of time, years even, to develop the strength they need to withstand the pounding for a race with the word *marathon* in the name.

SPEEDWORK

You're not ready to move up in distance, but you want to knock some time off the clock? See that finishing time a few minutes faster? That's what a few of our test panelists hoped for—and achieved. Roxy dropped her 5-K time to below 11 minutes per mile; Dorene knocked 7 minutes off her time between her first 5-K and her third. Talk about satisfying.

So if your 30-minute runs feel stale, try a speed workout once per week. Here are two workouts to try:

WORKOUT 1

- Run at your normal pace for the first 10 minutes.
- Pick up the pace for 10 minutes to a harder effort level. Instead of being able to speak in complete sentences, you're breathing more heavily, so you're able to get out only three or four words at a time. It's a faster pace, but you're in control. You don't want to push so hard that you feel like you want to fall over exhausted after the 10 minutes are finished.
- Finish by running at your normal pace for the last 10 minutes.

WORKOUT 2

- Run at your normal pace for the first 10 minutes.
- Alternate 1 minute of hard running with 1 minute of easy running for the next 10 minutes. You should feel a noticeable change in pace

for the minute-long hard segments, but they shouldn't be so fast that you can't complete five of them.

- Finish by running at your normal pace for the last 10 minutes.

Workout 1 is an introduction to "tempo running," and Workout 2 is a basic "interval workout." Those types of runs are staples of competitive runners' routines. You can learn more about them at runnersworld.com.

Budd's Buzz: "As you work up to 60 minutes of running, you'll notice an amazing jump in your fitness. That hour-long run will also be a monster calorie burner. Most important, by slowly building up the long run, you'll be giving your legs plenty of time to adapt to the added work, so you'll protect yourself from overuse injuries that tend to crop up when people increase their mileage too quickly."

STAY UPRIGHT!

Stand near the finish line of any race, from a 5-K on up, and you'll see some runners crossing the line all hunched over. It looks as if they're searching for loose change on the ground in front of them. They're lean, basically fit, and strong in the legs—but weak in the middle.

That's why core strength is so important. As you learn to run long distances, don't neglect your midsection, the muscles in your abdominals, sides, and back. They're the ones that hold you upright. With a strong trunk keeping you straight, you'll get more air in your lungs with every breath and move with a longer, steadier stride. In other words, a strong core can make you faster.

Here are six simple exercises for strengthening your core muscles. Aim to do these exercises three times a week. Every gym has stability balls, or you can buy one at a store like Target or Amazon.com for about $15.

Plank: Start by lying on the floor, propped up on your forearms. With your knees and feet together and keeping your elbows under your shoulders, lift your torso, legs, and hips in a straight line from head to heels. Hold for 10 seconds. Build up to 30 seconds.

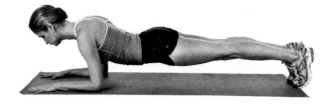

Side plank: Lie on your right side, supporting your upper body on your right forearm, with your left arm at your left side. Lift your hips off the floor, keeping your weight supported on the forearm and the side of your right foot. Put your left hand on your hip. Hold this position for

10 seconds and build up to 30. Switch sides and repeat. If this move is too difficult, start with your knees bent and support your weight on your knees instead of the side of your foot. (See photo at right below.)

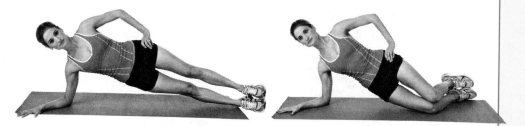

Superman: Yes, picture the superhero flying through the sky. Lie on your stomach with your arms extended in front of you and your legs straight. Raise your head, left arm, and right leg about 5 inches off the floor. Hold for 3 seconds, then lower. Repeat with your right arm and left leg. Build up to 10 repetitions on each side.

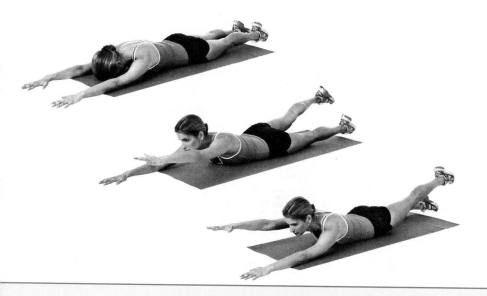

(continued on page 188)

Bridge: Lie on your back with your knees bent so your feet are flat on the floor. Keep your arms straight near your sides. Lift your hips and back off the floor until your body forms a straight line from your shoulders to your knees. Hold for 5 to 10 seconds. Lower yourself to the floor. Build up to 10 repetitions.

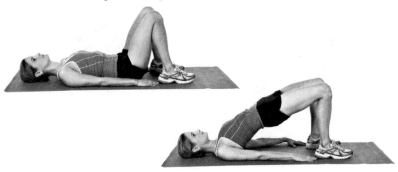

Abdominal curl: Sit on a stability ball with your knees shoulder-width apart and your feet flat on the floor. Walk your legs forward while leaning back until the ball is under your lower back. Place your hands on your shoulders or behind your head. Curl your upper body forward in a crunch motion, then return. You can alternate doing curls to the right and left sides to target the side muscles, which are called obliques. As you get stronger, increase the challenge to the obliques by moving your feet closer together.

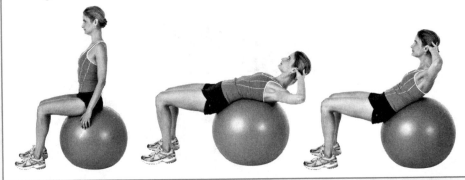

Body tuck: Lie facedown with your thighs on a stability ball and your hands on the floor in front of you so that your arms are perpendicular to your body. Slowly bring your legs toward your arms by bending your knees and letting the ball roll toward your shins. Pause, reverse the motion, and return to the starting position.

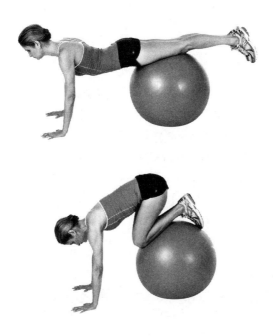

Fine-Tune It!

In this valedictory chapter, we want you to take a look back at the food changes you've made. What can you live with? What can't you live with? What was reasonable for you? What's going to help keep you on track for 7 good eating days a week, not just 5? What improvements can you tackle next?

COUNT IT AGAIN

Twelve weeks after you first tried a food log, it's a good time to try another one. You have extra pages at the back of this book. Use them to reexamine the patterns: where, why, and when you eat, as well as what you eat.

You might find that you're eating 200 calories less per day without even noticing. You might find that you're hungrier on your running days and you have to schedule your eating differently at those times.

Here's a page out of Dorene's food log when she was just beginning the program:

BEFORE FOOD LOG

TIME	FOOD	LOCATION	CALORIES
7:30 a.m.	Bowl of Special K with 1% milk	In front of computer	120
	2 cups of coffee with ¼ cup of 1% milk		110
11:45 a.m.	Tuna sandwich made with:	Kitchen table	167
	Hellman's mayo and relish		103
	1 slice of Kraft American cheese		70
	2 slices of split-top wheat bread		130
	Glass of 1% milk		100
2:30 p.m.	Starbucks medium caramel latte with whipped cream	In car	420
3:30 p.m.	½ apple and glass of water	Kitchen table	48

7:00 p.m.	8-oz steak	Kitchen table	390
	1/2 cup mushrooms		42
	6 spears of asparagus		20
	6 strawberries		23
	Glass of 1% milk		210
9:00 p.m.	5 Original Keebler's Club crackers	In front of TV	88
		Total calories:	2,041

AFTER FOOD LOG

TIME	FOOD	LOCATION	CALORIES
7:30 a.m.	Kashi GoLean Crunch with blueberries	Kitchen table	200
	Cup of coffee with fat-free milk and 1/2 packet Splenda		20
10:00 a.m.	Dunkin' Donuts medium coffee with fat-free milk and Splenda	Son's swimming practice	98
11:00 a.m.	Glass of water		0
12:30 p.m.	Deli turkey, 2 oz	Kitchen table	60
	Thin layer of Kraft light mayo		50
	1 slice of Kraft American cheese		70
	2 slices of Arnold's Bakery light 100% whole wheat bread		200
	4 celery sticks		1
	4 cherry tomatoes		20
	1 banana		105
	Glass of caffeine-free Diet Pepsi		0
4:15 p.m.	Zone Balance bar (honey nut)	Kitchen table	200
	1 apple		95
	Glass of water		0
7:30 p.m.	Glass of water		0
8:45 p.m.	6-inch Subway Sweet Onion Chicken Teriyaki sub with lettuce, onion, and sweet peppers	Kitchen table	381
	1 cup of fat-free milk		91
9:00 p.m.	Glass of water		0
		Total calories:	1,591

You can see where Dorene's doing better. She's whacked 450 calories from her day, which would get her close to losing a pound a week even before exercise. (She's one of those lucky people who says running actually suppresses her appetite.) She doesn't eat in front of the TV. She's avoiding the high-calorie pick-me-ups like the caramel latte, which accounts for 420 calories. She's getting plenty of fluids, so no problem on the 90 ounces she needs in a day. Her breakfast cereal has extra protein and fiber to fill her up, plus she's getting a serving of fruit in the morning now. She knows she has to go to her son's swim meet in the evening, so she has a late-afternoon snack and dinner when she gets home.

Are there still places where she could do better? Not many. Maybe a hard-ass dietitian would rather have her assembling her own sandwich at night with extra veggies instead of going to Subway. Who cares? Her day is busy. In Leslie's estimation, this day is just about perfect.

A word about Dorene: At the start, she was 193 pounds and needed 2,154 calories daily to maintain her weight. Now that she's dropped

Leslie's Lessons: "Cravings are more psychological than physiological unless you really have some sort of deficiency, which is rare. But if someone says, 'I'm just going to eat grapefruit,' chances are good that something else will be calling their name. And that could be a different texture—say, something crunchy, like a potato chip. Or a sweet baked good, because that's not the taste they're getting with the food they're eating. That's why I advise people to season their food and vary it in any way possible—different textures, tastes, temperatures, flavor profiles. The more variety, the less likely the craving for other items.

"A craving can also be due to external visual cues. You could have just eaten a meal, you're full, and you see the Oreo sitting there. It's not that you're hungry—it just looks good. So you have it. You can eliminate the cravings by not having those things sitting out. Get rid of the visual stimuli."

16 pounds, she has to run the numbers again. Her BMR has fallen to 1,495, and the total calories she needs in a day is 2,055, which is almost 100 less per day than when she started.

If you're running the numbers to create your own daily deficit, remember to recalculate every couple of months as the number on the scale shrinks. Personal Workbook Week 12 reminds you to do that math again.

UH-OH! HERE COME CRAVINGS!

You know what to eat, when to eat, how to eat, where to eat. Still, challenges crop up. Just when it has been a perfect day and week of eating, and you're starting to think you don't even miss junk food anymore, here comes a special cake at the office. Oh, great. Now what do I do?

When I find myself rummaging around at night seeking something chocolate and ultimately slipping my hand into the baking supplies for a handful of Nestle's semisweet chocolate chips, what's going on there? Is it a sign I'm not eating right? Am I not full enough?

Probably neither of those things, according to Leslie. I'm probably just bored with what's on the tube or with the "healthy" food I am eating.

Common Problems and Solutions

A diet with varied tastes and textures will help head off most cravings before they start. But what if I'm craving a second margarita while I'm out with friends or a second helping of potato salad at the family barbecue? Our lives are filled with challenges like these. Here, Leslie offers some suggestions for getting through the difficult times.

Problem: I'm going to happy hour on Friday with the gang from work.

Solution: This is a double whammy. Alcohol often gives people the munchies. And bar food is always fried. Eat a late-afternoon snack to take the edge off your hunger, preferably something with protein that will slow the alcohol's journey to the brain. Stand away from the beer nuts at the bar and order a lower-calorie drink, like a glass of wine or light beer, instead of a giant martini that could run 500 calories. A lot of people make the mistake of not realizing how much they really eat when they're at a bar. *It was just a few nibbles; it doesn't really count,* they think, then they pack in another good-size snack at home before bed. Be conscious of the calories from both the alcohol and the bar bites.

Problem: My toddler eats like a bird, and I end up eating all her food.

Solution: Kids don't require adult serving sizes, so try putting a lot less on her plate to start with. Then you won't feel bad about throwing out what she doesn't eat. Part of the reason kids are such selective eaters is that they're overwhelmed by what's put in front of them. Start with a tablespoon of each food you're serving. If she doesn't eat it, there's less for you to eat later. Or teach the kids to bring their own plate to the garbage can, scrape it, and put it next to the sink.

Problem: I'm about to fall asleep at my desk at 2:00 p.m., so I reach for a cookie.

Solution: Is it hunger or is it boredom? If it's boredom, stand up, take a walk around, and stop at the water fountain to get part of the 90 to 125 ounces of fluid you need in a day. If it's hunger, plan a healthy snack. Or divide your lunch in two parts. Eat half when you normally would and the other half when you hit your afternoon lull. That way you're getting through the problem period and you aren't adding unnecessary calories to the day.

Problem: We're having cake at the office. Just because it's Wednesday.

Solution: If you feel the need to have a piece of cake because it really is a special occasion, have it. Then make a compromise later in the day. Save the nuts and fruit you brought for a snack for tomorrow, since you've already had the cake. If your office is constantly stacked with treats, put them in the fridge with a sign on the front: "Goodies inside!" If it's not sitting out where you can see it, you'll be better able to resist.

Problem: The family barbecue this weekend means dogs, burgers, and Uncle Jeff's famous potato salad.

Solution: Make a good decision about what you're going to bring. Offer to contribute a fruit salad. Everyone loves it if they're not the ones cutting it up. Then enjoy the special foods that you don't get to eat regularly, like your uncle's potato salad, but stay away from everyday offerings like potato chips. They don't taste any different just because you're eating them at a family gathering.

THE FINE ART OF EATING OUT

I asked Leslie if she had any restaurants she'll never go to. And while she used to avoid fried-chicken places, pretty much any establishment these days has at least one reasonable offering, even KFC, which has a grilled chicken option. Still, navigating a restaurant meal without sabotaging your healthy-eating efforts can be tricky. Here's how to do it:

- Make special requests. Every business is competing for customers, and restaurants are no exception. They should be able to accommodate you when you ask for dressings and sauces "on the side." (Remember Meg Ryan's character in *When Harry Met Sally?* She terrorized waitresses with her "on the side" requests, but it turns out she was onto something. That movie came out in 1989.) A line chef can dump three times more salad dressing than you need on your salad. Ask for it on the side so you call the shots. If you're ordering Asian food, ask for it steamed with the sauce on the side, which you drizzle on.

- If you're trying to lose weight, steer clear of places that offer all-you-can-eat or automatic refills. It's just too darn tempting. *Bottomless* is not a good word for healthy eaters.

- Watch the bread before dinner. Ask the server not to bring the bread basket but, instead, to give you a small plate and a single piece of bread. If you're ravenous, request your salad as soon as you sit down. The establishment should be eager to please you. (If not, go somewhere else next time.)

- Salad bars can be great as long as you avoid the Waldorf salad and creamy macaroni. Take advantage of all the things that you normally wouldn't chop for yourself and make a colorful plate.

- Eating out is an indulgence. We want to feel spoiled, so go ahead and order something you wouldn't normally make for yourself. A petite filet mignon is only 6 ounces. Great, have it! Ask the server to hold the melted butter on top, though. And if the starch choices aren't appealing, ask for extra vegetables instead.

- If you're making a rare visit to a restaurant famous for a fabulous dessert, have the fabulous dessert! Just skip the baked potato or the rice pilaf. Leslie reminds us that no one ever walks out of a restaurant saying, "That was the best baked potato I ever had." Rice pilaf is rarely memorable. Plan what it is you really want, then bargain accordingly.

ASK YOURSELF WHAT WORKS AND DO MORE OF IT

The test panel was pretty honest about the changes they could live with and the changes they couldn't abide. Brutally honest, in fact. Here's what Donna, 50, told me about breakfast and eating in the car:

> I have been a cereal eater for breakfast for a long time, but I changed that after learning more about the importance of protein. I started to eat a protein bar for breakfast instead. I know I'm not supposed to eat in the car, but I have a 45-minute commute in the morning. So I eat the protein bar with my coffee and a banana while I'm driving. I have all the time in the world to eat slowly, but if I ate breakfast at home I would be rushing. I find that the protein bar and banana, consumed slowly, keep me satisfied until lunch. So you can't say that it's *always* bad to eat in the car.

Point well taken, Donna. Sometimes the various bits of advice—like eating slowly, spacing your food intake, managing more fruits and vegeta-

FOOD TALK   Think It Through!

If there's one point we've wanted to get across in this book, it's that losing weight permanently requires some thought. You have to examine your eating and exercise habits almost as if you're an impartial observer. Then you can make changes, understand why you're making them, and stick with them.

> You have to examine your eating and exercise habits almost as if you're an impartial observer.

bles and protein—can't all be accomplished at once. So rank habits in order of importance and convenience to you, and attack them one at a time.

EXERCISE YOUR MIND

People say to Leslie all the time, "I don't know why I'm not losing weight." If you bring your mind to the game and take an honest look at what you're doing, you'll have the answers.

Only by creating a calorie deficit can you lose weight. By now you've learned that you have to exercise more, eat less, or do both. Along the way, you've found answers to some critical questions: How many calories are in this food? How big is that serving? How much good is this workout doing?

In Leslie's experience helping clients lose weight, she has noticed that the self-education process takes about 12 weeks. In other words, you need 3 months to train your brain to make good behaviors habitual. You need 3 months to learn to do the flip-and-read on the labels at the grocery store. To learn how to plan and shop. To learn how to eat the right balance

Leslie's Lessons: "Lose the negative self-talk! People start thinking that they've eaten a forbidden food and they'll never be able to change. Eating a certain food doesn't make you a good or bad person.

"Remember to tackle not just the food items but your thoughts, too. Try saying this to yourself: *Maybe my day wasn't perfect. It's okay. I'll try again later. I'll move on.*"

of protein and carbohydrate, with sufficient vitamins from fruits and vegetables mixed in. It takes a substantial period of time to evaluate your habits, see where you're adding extra calories that you don't need, change the behavior, and make the changes stick.

According to Budd, it takes about the same amount of time—12 weeks—to turn a person into a runner. Funny how that works, right?

All these tips and lessons and calorie calculations are not meant to make eating a joyless exercise. And we're not saying that every single bite that goes into your mouth for the rest of your life has to be obsessively logged and counted. No one is denying that food is comfort and that eating can be emotional.

This eating plan is in no way meant to deprive you of the foods you love most. We hope you've seen along the way that the suggestions in *RYBO* are just that—suggestions. There's nothing rigid in here, nothing strictly forbidden. The point is to develop an understanding of the calories in the food you eat, how those foods affect your calorie total for the day, and how that number makes you maintain, gain, or lose weight. Your brain has to come to the table with you.

Finally, we hope *RYBO* has helped you escape the rigid way you view yourself. No more "good" or "bad." Instead, you're a work in progress, as an eater and an athlete.

Move on. Make better choices at the next meal, put your sneakers on, and keep going.

SECRETS OF THE TEST PANEL

JULIE, 38

Job: Processing manager for a real estate agency; mother of two

Goals: To participate in a local 5-K and look better

Starting weight: 181 pounds

Ending weight: 168 pounds

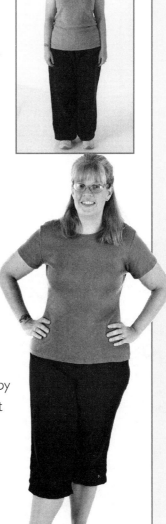

Back in the Day: I'd try to run and I'd find myself breathing *extremely* hard. That's not fun. But walking wasn't getting me too far with my weight-loss goals.

Building Up: Once I got my breathing down, because I was going so slowly, it was pretty easy to increase my time. But I had trouble with going from 14 minutes of running to 30 minutes straight. So I did 19 minutes of running. Then 23 minutes of running. It worked for me.

Music Makes the Run: You wouldn't know by looking at me, but I'm a rocker. I can't work out without it. Have to have my Metallica and Kid Rock and my eighties' hair bands—Bon Jovi, Cinderella, Poison, and Ratt.

Appendix A

Additional Resources for Running and Weight Loss

Leslie's 12 Rules for Weight-Loss Success

1. **Log it!** Write down everything you eat for 1 week. A log gives you an unflinching look at your calorie consumption. With this record, you can examine your habits to see what eating patterns are sabotaging your weight-loss efforts.

2. **Space it!** Eat at regular 4- to 5-hour intervals throughout the day. Don't wait to eat until you're starving, but you do need to give your body some time off from eating during the day. The strategy of "grazing" often does not work for people trying to lose weight. Eat breakfast every day. An evening snack can be fine, especially if you eat dinner early, stay up late, or work out in the evening.

3. **Measure it!** Leave your measuring spoons and cups out so you remember to use them. Get in the habit of measuring cereal, rice and pasta, juice, salad dressing, and other items that don't come in single-serving sizes. Often we allot ourselves much more than a serving. It takes a while to train the eyes and brain to recognize what a real serving size is.

4. **Shop it!** Plan a week's worth of meals, check what ingredients you have on hand, and make a comprehensive shopping list. When you get to the store, stick to your list. This will save you time and money. If you load your cart with a mix of nutrient-rich foods, including produce, low-fat dairy products, lean meats, and whole grains, the cart won't have room for junk food.

5. **Slow it down!** Chew your food and taste it. Put your fork down between bites. Turn off the TV so you're concentrating on your meal. Talk to your mealtime companions. Try to take 20 minutes per meal. This gives the nerve endings in the digestive tract enough time to signal the brain that you're full. Slowing down prevents overeating.

6. Color it! Add one red, yellow, orange, green, or purple food to every meal. Making sure you get fruits or vegetables with each meal will help give your body the vitamins, minerals, and fiber it needs. You'll also feel fuller.

7. Muscle it! Eat some protein at every meal. Aim to get ½ gram of protein per pound of body weight in a day. Protein preserves and builds muscle mass and makes you feel satisfied. And your body works harder digesting protein, which burns more calories.

8. Drink it! Women need 90 ounces of fluid each day; men need 125 ounces. As long as it's not alcohol, any liquid counts toward the total. Drink a glass of water with every meal, but coffee, tea, broth, and even the liquid in fruits and vegetables contribute to the fluid you need.

9. Swap it! Look for healthy swaps you can make, like buying bread with more fiber and selecting lower-fat dairy and leaner meat. These painless swaps can cut calories and add more nutrients to your diet.

10. Season it! Honor your taste buds. Using herbs, spices, seasoning mixes, and flavorings is an easy way to give healthy foods an extra kick. If your mouth gets bored, you're more likely to experience cravings, which can sabotage your healthy eating.

11. Fine-tune it! Log your food intake again and figure out what parts of your diet have improved—and where you still need to devote some attention.

12. Think it through! Anticipate those situations, like restaurant dining or weekend events, that might challenge your resolve to eat well. Plan for how you can enjoy special occasions without overeating. Examine your mind-set and avoid the "I've blown it" mentality. People get into trouble when they feel like a large meal or unhealthy treat wrecks their diet, so they might as well continue to overeat throughout the day. Instead, acknowledge that you've eaten more than you wanted on that one occasion, move on, and try to do better the rest of the day.

Budd's 12 Stages of
Running for Beginners

Repeat each workout at least three or four times in a week before moving on to the next stage.

Stage 1: Build up to 30 minutes of nonstop walking.

Stage 2: Walk for 4 minutes. Run for 1 minute. Repeat that sequence four more times. End with 4 minutes of walking.
> **Total workout time: 29 minutes, 5 of which are running.**

Stage 3: Walk for 4 minutes. Run for 2 minutes. Repeat that sequence four more times. End with 3 minutes of walking.
> **Total workout time: 33 minutes, 10 of which are running.**

Stage 4: Walk for 3 minutes. Run for 3 minutes. Repeat that sequence four more times. End with 3 minutes of walking.
> **Total workout time: 33 minutes, 15 of which are running.**

Stage 5: Walk for 2 minutes 30 seconds. Run for 5 minutes. Repeat that sequence three more times. End with 3 minutes of walking.
> **Total workout time: 33 minutes, 20 of which are running.**

Stage 6: Walk for 3 minutes. Run for 7 minutes. Repeat that sequence two more times. End with 3 minutes of walking.
> **Total workout time: 33 minutes, 21 of which are running.**

Stage 7: Walk for 2 minutes. Run for 8 minutes. Repeat that sequence two more times. End with 3 minutes of walking.
   Total workout time: 33 minutes, 24 of which are running.

Stage 8: Walk for 2 minutes. Run for 9 minutes. Repeat that sequence one more time. Then walk for 2 minutes, run for 8 minutes. End with 3 minutes of walking.
   Total workout time: 35 minutes, 26 of which are running.

Stage 9: Walk for I minute. Run for 9 minutes. Repeat that sequence two more times. End with 3 minutes of walking.
   Total workout time: 33 minutes, 27 of which are running.

Stage 10: Walk for 2 minutes. Run for 13 minutes. Repeat that sequence one more time. End with 3 minutes of walking.
   Total workout time: 33 minutes, 26 of which are running.

Stage II: Walk for 2 minutes. Run for 14 minutes. Then walk for I minute, run for 14 minutes. End with 3 minutes of walking.
   Total workout time: 34 minutes, 28 of which are running.

Stage 12: Walk for 3 minutes (or until you're good and ready). Then run for 30 minutes nonstop. End with 3 minutes of walking.
   Total workout time: 36 minutes, 30 of which are running.

Appendix B

Your Personal
Workbook

How to Use Your Personal Workbook

Progress! Moving toward a goal! Success! Here's a place to keep track of it all. This workbook is meant to help you note your achievements, record your thoughts, and see what's working well (and maybe not quite so well) for you.

At the most basic level, this is a place for you to **record your weight each week.** If you want to leave it at that, fine. You've got a private spot to jot down the number the scale shows each week. Our hope is that you'll see the numbers moving in the right direction.

We're also providing space for you to **write down your workouts,** including the places you run and your thoughts on how running feels. If you want to, you can record your running and weight-loss goals and include the names of the people with whom you've shared your ambitions. We've thrown out a few probing questions to get you to think about what exercise is doing for you. When you understand how you're feeling, you might find you're more motivated to get out the door three or four times a week.

The **Food Talk** sections of the workbook review the tips in the book, such as the advice about serving sizes and timing your meals. As you're analyzing your eating habits and food choices, you might realize some things about yourself, things like "Hey, I always eat in front of my computer" or "A serving of granola is a lot smaller than a serving of Cheerios."

Readers willing to take the extra step and **learn more about weight-loss math** can use this workbook to go through those calculations. You don't need anything more than a calculator for simple addition, subtraction, and multiplication, so don't be intimidated if numbers aren't your strong suit.

You can calculate how many calories your body needs to maintain its current weight. You can count how many calories you're consuming and see how many calories walking and running will burn. The chapters in this book give the complete explanations for these calculations. If you've skipped ahead to this workbook and something has you confused, go back and read the chapter on that topic. If that doesn't answer your question, drop a line to Sarah@runyourbuttoffbook.com.

Not everyone wants to crunch the numbers, and we know that. But our experts, dietitian Leslie Bonci and coach Budd Coates, know that a little bit of information can be a powerful tool. Armed with knowledge about your own body and your own habits, you can develop a plan for training and weight loss that will work. Why? Because it's all yours.

Personal Workbook Week 1

Making the Numbers Work for You

Date:	Weight this week:

STAGE 1 WORKOUT

- Build up to 30 minutes of nonstop walking.
  Do this workout four times in 1 week.

Enter the days you plan to work out this week. Mark Y or N if you finished the exercise on that day. Enter the details of the workout and any impressions.

I plan to walk on the following days:	DID YOU DO IT (Y/N)?	WALK TIME:	TOTAL WORKOUT TIME:
Date: Time:			
Date: Time:			
Date: Time:			
Date: Time:			

Thoughts on the workouts: weather, effort level, aches and pains, challenges, successes. How hard did it feel?

1
2
3
4

Thoughts on location: Just right? Too hilly? Too crowded? Drinking fountain or facilities available? Would you go back?

1
2
3
4

Your Starting Stats

Height:		Weight:	
Chest:	Waist:	Hips:	Thighs:

Weigh yourself first thing in the morning, after you've used the bathroom, clothes off.

Take your measurements. Hold a tape measure around yourself at the chest, waist, hips, and thighs. The tape measure should be snug against your body but not so tight that you're cutting off your circulation. (Men, you only need to measure your waist.)

Weight-Loss Math
How Much Do You Need to Eat to Stay the Same Weight?
This calculation figures out your basal metabolic rate, the calories your body needs in a day for all the basic functions that keep you alive. To do it, you need your weight, height, gender, and age. You can do this online using the *Runner's World* calculator at www.runnersworld.com/rybo.

Or calculate it here using the Harris-Benedict equation.

For women:

Take your weight in pounds and multiply it by 4.3: _____

Take your height in inches and multiply it by 4.7: _____

Add those two numbers together: _____

Then add 655: _____

This gives you subtotal A: _____

Now take your age and multiply it by 4.7: _____

This gives you subtotal B: _____

Now subtract subtotal B from subtotal A: _____

This is your BMR.

For men, the equation is different:

Take your weight in pounds and multiply it by 6.3: _____

Take your height in inches and multiply it by 12.9: _____

Add those two numbers together: _____

Then add 66: _____

This gives you subtotal A: _____

Now take your age and multiply it by 6.8: _____

This gives you subtotal B: _____

Now subtract subtotal B from subtotal A: _____

This is your BMR.

Example: a woman who is 140 pounds, 5 feet 5 inches, and 40 years old

Weight (140) × 4.3 = 602

Height in inches (65) × 4.7 = 305.5

Add those two numbers together, then add 655.

Subtotal A = 1,562.5

Age (40) × 4.7 = 188

Subtotal B = 188

Subtotal A (1,562.5) − Subtotal B (188) = 1,374.5 calories

Example: a man who is 180 pounds, 5 feet 10 inches, and 45 years old

Weight (180) × 6.3 = 1,134

Height in inches (70) × 12.9 = 903

Add those two numbers together, then add 66.

Subtotal A = 2,103

Age (45) × 6.8 = 306

Subtotal B = 306

Subtotal A (2,103) − Subtotal B (306) = 1,797 calories

Total Calories You Need to Maintain Your Current Weight

Now calculate the calories you use in a day, not including formal exercise.

If you are sedentary, multiply your BMR x 1.2.

If you are lightly active, multiply your BMR x 1.375.

If you are moderately active, multiply your BMR x 1.55.

If you are very active, multiply your BMR x 1.725.

If you are extra active, multiply your BMR x 1.9.

Enter the number here: _____

This is the total number of calories you need in a day, before formal exercise, to maintain your current weight. Eat more than this and you'll gain weight. Burn more calories with exercise or eat less than this, and you'll lose weight.

What do you think? Is the total more than you expected or less than you expected?

Personal Workbook Week 2

Making the Numbers Work for You

Date:	Weight this week:

STAGE 2 WORKOUT

- Walk for 4 minutes. Run for I minute.

- Repeat that sequence four more times.

- End with 4 minutes of walking.

Total workout time: 29 minutes, 5 of which are running.

Do this workout at least three or four times in a week
before moving on to the next stage.

Enter the days you plan to work out this week. Mark Y or N if you finished the exercise on that day. Enter the details of the workout and any impressions.

I plan to workout on the following days:	DID YOU DO IT (Y/N)?	WALK TIME	RUN TIME	TOTAL WORKOUT TIME
Date: Time:				
Date: Time:				
Date: Time:				
Date: Time:				

Thoughts on the workouts: weather, effort level, aches and pains, challenges, successes. How hard did it feel?

1	
2	
3	
4	

Additional exercise during the week: (Examples: yoga, swimming, dog walking, etc.)

HOW TO USE THE FOOD LOG

Writing down everything you eat for a week will help you achieve your weight-loss goals. If you log honestly, you'll get an accurate picture of what, when, where, and how much you consume. With that information in front of you, you'll be able to make a realistic plan for cutting back and shedding pounds. Here's a bit of the food log to start with, and you can find additional pages starting on page 250.

TIME	WHERE ARE YOU EATING?	WHAT ARE YOU EATING?

At first glance, I learned that I eat well at these times:

Day   Date

HOW MUCH ARE YOU EATING?	ARE YOU HUNGRY (H) or NOT HUNGRY (NH)?	RATE YOUR DAY 1–5 1—Bad day 5—Great day

At first glance, I learned that these times are problematic for me:

Personal Workbook Week 3

Making the Numbers Work for You

Date:	Weight this week:

STAGE 3 WORKOUT

- Walk for 4 minutes. Run for 2 minutes.
- Repeat that sequence four more times.
- End with 3 minutes of walking.

Total workout time: 33 minutes, 10 of which are running.

Do this workout at least three or four times in a week before moving on to the next stage.

Enter the days you plan to work out this week. Mark Y or N if you finished the exercise on that day. Enter the details of the workout and any impressions.

I plan to workout on the following days:	DID YOU DO IT (Y/N)?	WALK TIME	RUN TIME	TOTAL WORKOUT TIME
Date: Time:				
Date: Time:				
Date: Time:				
Date: Time:				

Thoughts on the workouts: weather, effort level, aches and pains, challenges, successes. How hard did it feel?

1	
2	
3	
4	

Additional exercise during the week:

Food Talk: Spacing Your Food Intake

Look at the food log you started last week. Are you eating at regular intervals throughout the day and eating about the same amount of food each time? If not, when are you eating too much? When are you eating too little?

Here are my problem times and my plans for leveling out my food intake:

Goal Setting

Take some time to think about your goals. They can be about running, racing, weight, health, even energy level. Consider: What do you really want for yourself? How do you envision yourself in the future? How hard are you willing to work to get there?

If weight loss is a goal, remember the guidelines set forth by the National Institutes of Health. A reasonable rate of weight loss, which ensures you're losing fat and not muscle or water weight, is between ½ and 1 pound per week. Keep that in mind and set realistic goals.

GOAL	DEADLINE FOR MEETING IT	HOW WILL YOU KNOW WHEN YOU'VE ACHIEVED YOUR GOAL?
1.		
2.		
3.		
4.		
5.		
Three people I'm going to tell about my goals:		
1.		
2.		
3.		

Personal Workbook Week 4

Making the Numbers Work for You

Date:	Weight this week:

STAGE 4 WORKOUT

- Walk for 3 minutes. Run for 3 minutes.
- Repeat that sequence four more times.
- End with 3 minutes of walking.

Total workout time: 33 minutes, 15 of which are running.

Do this workout at least three or four times in a week before moving on to the next stage.

Enter the days you plan to work out this week. Mark Y or N if you finished the exercise on that day. Enter the details of the workout and any impressions.

I plan to workout on the following days:	DID YOU DO IT (Y/N)?	WALK TIME	RUN TIME	TOTAL WORKOUT TIME
Date: Time:				
Date: Time:				
Date: Time:				
Date: Time:				

Thoughts on the workouts: weather, effort level, aches and pains, challenges, successes. How hard did it feel?

1	
2	
3	
4	

At this point you're running and walking in equal intervals. How does this feel?

How do you feel when people see you running? Proud? Embarrassed? Indifferent?

Additional exercise during the week:

Food Talk: Measure Everything!

Leave your measuring cups and spoons out, and remember to measure your serving sizes, especially for cereal, rice, pasta, juice, and sweets.

Have you been surprised at serving sizes this week? Did you discover that you've been eating more than one serving of any foods? Maybe you were happy to find that certain foods allow more than you realized.

These are the foods I have to be careful with:

Weight-Loss Math: Making a Plan for Weight Loss

When you examine how many calories you're eating each day and how many calories you're burning each day through exercise, you can make a blueprint for weight loss. This section takes you through those steps.

This might seem like a lot of number crunching, but if you go through the process, you can determine what exercising and eating do for your weight. You'll be able to rely on data instead of guesswork.

The first step is to find out how many calories you are currently eating. Go back and look at the food log you compiled in Personal Workbook Week 2, and calculate the calories in each of the foods you recorded. Sites like MyPyramid.gov, CalorieKing.com, and FitDay.com can help you total the calories in the foods you're eating.

Count for at least 1 day and write the numbers below. Or count for a few days and take the average.

Date: _____   **Total calories today:** _____

To lose ½ pound a week, you need to cut 250 calories per day by eating less or exercising more. To lose 1 pound a week, you need to cut 500 calories per day through a combination of diet and exercise.

What times during the day would it be realistic to cut back your calorie consumption? Breakfast, lunch, or dinner? Snacks? Nighttime eating? Alcohol consumption? List a few times and meals when you can cut your caloric intake.

I PLAN TO MAKE HEALTHIER CHOICES AT:	NUMBER OF CALORIES THIS WILL CUT:
1.	
2.	
3.	

Exercise Plan

How many times can you count on exercising in a week? Be realistic.

I have been walking and running _____ times for _____ minutes each time.

To get an accurate sense of your calorie burn during a typical workout, you need to know your distance. Try one workout on a measured course or around a track so you know how far you're going.

Take your body weight and multiply it by 0.53 to get the number of calories burned each time you walk 1 mile. Take your body weight and multiply it by 0.75 to get the number of calories you burn running 1 mile.

Weight _____ x 0.53 x _____ miles walked = _____ calories burned walking

Weight _____ x 0.75 x _____ miles run = _____ calories burned running

Add the two together: _____

Average workout burns _____ calories, multiplied by _____ workouts per week.

Weekly calorie deficit (calories saved from eating + calories burned while exercising): _____

Take that number and divide it by 3,500: _____

This will result in weight loss of _____ pounds per week.

> **Example: A 180-pound woman decides to cut 200 calories from her eating each day, or 1,400 calories a week. She also runs and walks four times a week, 2 miles each time (1 mile walking and 1 mile running).**
>
> 180 pounds x 0.53 x 1 mile = 95.4 calories burned walking
>
> 180 pounds x 0.75 x 1 mile = 135 calories burned running
>
> She burns 230 calories per workout, or 920 calories per week.
>
> Combined with cutting 1,400 calories from her diet each week, she's creating a weekly deficit of 2,320 calories. Divide by 3,500 and you get 0.66. This will help her lose ⅔ pound per week.

Personal Workbook Week 5

Making the Numbers Work for You

Date:	Weight this week:

STAGE 5 WORKOUT

- Walk for 2 minutes and 30 seconds. Run for 5 minutes.
- Repeat that sequence three more times.
- End with 3 minutes of walking.

Total workout time: 33 minutes, 20 of which are running.

Do this workout at least three or four times in a week before moving on to the next stage.

Enter the days you plan to work out this week. Mark Y or N if you finished the exercise on that day. Enter the details of the workout and any impressions.

I plan to workout on the following days:	DID YOU DO IT (Y/N)?	WALK TIME	RUN TIME	TOTAL WORKOUT TIME
Date: Time:				
Date: Time:				
Date: Time:				
Date: Time:				

Thoughts on the workouts: weather, effort level, aches and pains, challenges, successes. How hard did it feel?

1	
2	
3	
4	

In Stage 5, the workout shifts so you spend more time running than walking. How does this feel?

Feel ready to sign up for a race? If so, which one? If not, are there any nearby races that you can go watch?

Who's on your support team? Are they checking in with you?

Food Talk: Supermarket Strategies
Good eating starts at the grocery store. For menu planning ideas and shopping tips, go back and read *RYBO* Chapter 5.

Planning Dinner This Week:

	MY PLAN	DID YOU STICK TO IT (Y/N)?
Monday		
Tuesday		
Wednesday		
Thursday		
Friday		
Saturday		
Sunday		

Personal Workbook Week 6

Making the Numbers Work for You

Date:	Weight this week:

STAGE 6 WORKOUT

- Walk for 3 minutes. Run for 7 minutes.
- Repeat that sequence two more times.
- End with 3 minutes of walking.

Total workout time: 33 minutes, 21 of which are running.

Do this workout at least three or four times in a week before moving on to the next stage.

Enter the days you plan to work out this week. Mark Y or N if you finished the workout on that day. Enter the details of the exercise and any impressions.

I plan to workout on the following days:	DID YOU DO IT (Y/N)?	WALK TIME	RUN TIME	TOTAL WORKOUT TIME
Date: Time:				
Date: Time:				
Date: Time:				
Date: Time:				

Thoughts on the workouts: weather, effort level, aches and pains, challenges, successes. How hard did it feel?

1	
2	
3	
4	

Food Talk: Slow It Down

Find time this week to linger over a meal. Or see if you can adjust your schedule so you're sharing more meals with family or friends instead of eating on the fly. Record your observations. Do you eat more or less when you eat slowly?

Take a moment to record your thoughts on treats and food "rewards." Are you tempted to eat more after a long workout? When are your most vulnerable times? Can you plan for sensible treats, or do your indulgences catch you off guard?

Personal Workbook Week 7

Making the Numbers Work for You

Date:	Weight this week:

STAGE 7 WORKOUT

- Walk for 2 minutes. Run for 8 minutes.

- Repeat that sequence two more times.

- End with 3 minutes of walking.

Total workout time: 33 minutes, 24 of which are running.

Do this workout at least three or four times in a week
before moving on to the next stage.

Enter the days you plan to work out this week. Mark Y or N if you finished the exercise on that day. Enter the details of the workout and any impressions.

I plan to workout on the following days:	DID YOU DO IT (Y/N)?	WALK TIME	RUN TIME	TOTAL WORKOUT TIME
Date: Time:				
Date: Time:				
Date: Time:				
Date: Time:				

Thoughts on the workouts: weather, effort level, aches and pains, challenges, successes. How hard did it feel?

1	
2	
3	
4	

Additional exercise during the week:

Eight minutes is a long time to run. Do you count every passing minute or is your mind starting to wander during the running portions?

Food Talk: Color It!

Add one fruit or vegetable to every meal. What have you tried?

FRUIT/VEGETABLE	MEAL	HOW WAS IT?
1.		
2.		
3.		

Postworkout Hunger Level

How would you rate your appetite after a run/walk workout? Are you hungrier than usual? About the same? Or not hungry at all?

Goals Update:

One month later, let's check the goals you set for yourself in Week 3 of this workbook.

GOAL	DEADLINE FOR MEETING IT	MET GOAL/ STILL IN PROGRESS
1.		
2		
3.		
4.		
5.		

If you've met any of your goals, think about some new ones:

GOAL	DEADLINE FOR MEETING IT	HOW WILL YOU KNOW WHEN YOU'VE ACHIEVED YOUR GOAL?
6.		
7.		
8.		

Personal Workbook Week 8

Making the Numbers Work for You

Date:	Weight this week:

STAGE 8 WORKOUT

- Walk for 2 minutes. Run for 9 minutes.

- Repeat that sequence one more time.

- Then walk for 2 minutes, run for 8 minutes.

- End with 3 minutes of walking.

Total workout time: 35 minutes, 26 of which are running.

Do this workout at least three or four times in a week
before moving on to the next stage.

Enter the days you plan to work out this week. Mark Y or N if you finished the exercise on that day. Enter the details of the workout and any impressions.

I plan to workout on the following days:	DID YOU DO IT (Y/N)?	WALK TIME	RUN TIME	TOTAL WORKOUT TIME
Date: Time:				
Date: Time:				
Date: Time:				
Date: Time:				

Thoughts on the workouts: weather, effort level, aches and pains, challenges, successes. How hard did it feel?

1	
2	
3	
4	

Additional exercise during the week:

Food Talk: Meeting Your Protein Needs

Protein is a vitally important component of your diet; *RYBO* explains why in Chapter 8. Aim for 0.5 gram of protein per pound of body weight. Use your goal weight in this calculation.

Example: A woman currently weighs 180 pounds and hopes to drop to 160 pounds. She should be getting at least 80 grams of protein (160 pounds × 0.5 gram) per day.

One day this week, log your food intake again. Tally the grams of protein in each food. See how you're doing against your target intake.

	PROTEIN (IN GRAMS)	CALORIES
Breakfast		
Lunch		
Dinner		
Snacks		
TOTAL		
TARGET		

The Weekend Trap

It's more challenging to stick to healthy eating resolutions on the weekend than it is during the week. Write down your biggest weekend challenges and how you plan to meet them.

Weight-Loss Math

As your workouts shift to include more running, the calorie burn from each workout increases as well. Let's look at the calculation you did in Week 4 of this workbook to see how many more calories you are burning now that your workouts are more intense.

To get an accurate sense of your calorie burn for a typical workout, you need to know your distance. Try one workout on a measured course or around a track so you know how far you're going.

Take your body weight and multiply it by 0.53 to get the number of calories burned each time you walk 1 mile. Take your body weight and multiply it by 0.75 to get the number of calories you burn running 1 mile.

Weight _____ × 0.53 × _____ miles walked = _____ calories burned walking

Weight _____ × 0.75 × _____ miles run = _____ calories burned running

Add the two together: _____

Average workout burns _____ calories, multiplied by _____ workouts per week.

In comparison, look back at Week 4 of this workbook. How many calories was the average workout burning then? Enter the number here: _____

Personal Workbook Week 9

Making the Numbers Work for You

Date:	Weight this week:

STAGE 9 WORKOUT

- Walk for 1 minute. Run for 9 minutes.

- Repeat that sequence two more times.

- End with 3 minutes of walking.

Total workout time: 33 minutes, 27 of which are running.

Do this workout at least three or four times in a week before moving on to the next stage.

Enter the days you plan to work out this week. Mark Y or N if you finished the exercise on that day. Enter the details of the workout and any impressions.

I plan to workout on the following days:	DID YOU DO IT (Y/N)?	WALK TIME	RUN TIME	TOTAL WORKOUT TIME
Date: Time:				
Date: Time:				
Date: Time:				
Date: Time:				

Thoughts on the workouts: weather, effort level, aches and pains, challenges, successes. How hard did it feel?

1	
2	
3	
4	

Additional activity this week:

Treasure the compliments: Has anyone seen you running? Commented on your discipline? Noticed any weight loss? Record the compliments and enjoy them all over again.

Food Talk: Make Healthy Swaps

When you're watching your weight, you can make healthy swaps or pick better-for-you versions of food to save a few calories. Dairy and meat should be lower in fat; bread should be higher in fiber. It takes some experimenting to find brands you like. Review *RYBO* Chapter 9 for more ideas. List a few swaps—foods you can do without and their substitutes you can live with.

1. I tried replacing _____ with _____.

2. I tried replacing _____ with _____.

3. I tried replacing _____ with _____.

Personal Workbook Week 10

Making the Numbers Work for You

Date:	Weight this week:

STAGE 10 WORKOUT

- Walk for 2 minutes. Run for 13 minutes.

- Repeat that sequence one more time.

- End with 3 minutes of walking.

Total workout time: 33 minutes, 26 of which are running.
Do this workout at least three or four times in a week
before moving on to the next stage.

Enter the days you plan to work out this week. Mark Y or N if you finished the exercise on that day. Enter the details of the workout and any impressions.

I plan to workout on the following days:	DID YOU DO IT (Y/N)?	WALK TIME	RUN TIME	TOTAL WORKOUT TIME
Date: Time:				
Date: Time:				
Date: Time:				
Date: Time:				

Thoughts on the workouts: weather, effort level, aches and pains, challenges, successes. How hard did it feel?

1
2
3
4

Additional exercise during the week:

Running for 13 minutes is a significant amount of time—close to a mile for some people, more than a mile for others. How did you feel?

Food Talk: Variety Matters!

When you are trying to lose weight, it's easy to get stuck in a "food rut" and eat the same things over and over again. But when your taste buds get bored, you're more likely to overdo it when given the opportunity. Try varying your food routine. Mix up the flavors with herbs and spices, change where you eat, even replace the plate you're using—anything to keep it interesting.

This week I varied my eating habits in these ways:

1.
2.
3.

How much hunger are you feeling?

Try to eat before you're famished. The converse is also true: Stop eating before you're stuffed. If you have problems with portion control, try serving yourself a plate with 25 percent less food on it. Remember to eat slowly. Record your impressions of hunger, fullness, and eating 25 percent less here.

1. I'm most hungry at:
2. I'm most likely to overeat at:
3. If I serve myself a smaller amount of food, what happens?

Personal Workbook Week 11

Making the Numbers Work for You

Date:	Weight this week:

STAGE 11 WORKOUT

- Walk for 2 minutes. Run for 14 minutes.

- Then walk for 1 minute. Run for 14 minutes.

- End with 3 minutes of walking.

Total workout time: 34 minutes, 28 of which are running.
Do this workout at least three or four times in a week
before moving on to the next stage.

Enter the days you plan to work out this week. Mark Y or N if you finished the exercise on that day. Enter the details of the workout and any impressions.

I plan to workout on the following days:	DID YOU DO IT (Y/N)?	WALK TIME	RUN TIME	TOTAL WORKOUT TIME
Date: Time:				
Date: Time:				
Date: Time:				
Date: Time:				

Thoughts on the workouts: weather, effort level, aches and pains, challenges, successes. How hard did it feel?)

1
2
3
4

Additional exercise during the week:

How does the 1 minute of walking in the middle of the workout feel? Is it a minute of rest you need, or does it feel more difficult to stop and get started again?

Food Talk: Cravings and Problem Times

Do you have food cravings that are hard to resist? If so, for what? Can you find a way to satisfy your cravings with a small serving? Can you sacrifice something else to keep your calorie total in check? What are some trade-offs you can make?

What are your problem situations or times of the day? For instance, it could be the weekend, happy hour with coworkers, the midafternoon lull, or restaurant meals. Take account of your problem eating times, and make a plan for how you'll approach them the next time.

PROBLEM TIME	SOLUTION
1.	
2.	
3.	

Personal Workbook Week 12

Making the Numbers Work for You

Date:	Weight this week:

STAGE 12 WORKOUT

- Walk for 3 minutes (or until you're good and ready).
- Run for 30 minutes.
- End with 3 minutes of walking.

Total workout time: 36 minutes, 30 of which are running.
Repeat this sequence throughout your whole life.

Enter the days you plan to work out this week. Mark Y or N if you finished the exercise on that day. Enter the details of the workout and any impressions.

I plan to workout on the following days:	DID YOU DO IT (Y/N)?	WALK TIME	RUN TIME	TOTAL WORKOUT TIME
Date: Time:				
Date: Time:				
Date: Time:				
Date: Time:				

Thoughts on the workouts: weather, effort level, aches and pains, challenges, successes. How hard did it feel?

1	
2	
3	
4	

Additional exercise during the week:

Thirty minutes of running:

How did it feel? Did you celebrate your success? Did you tell anyone? Describe what happened the first time you ran for 30 minutes without stopping.

Weight-Loss Math: New Numbers for a Different Body

As you lose weight, the number of calories you burn in a day drops, too. So the BMR you calculated back in Week 1 of this workbook is probably out of date by now. Time to calculate it again.

Start by figuring out your basal metabolic rate, the calories your body needs in a day for all the basic functions that keep you alive. To do so, you need your weight, height, gender, and age.

You can do this online using the *Runner's World* calculator at www.runnersworld.com/rybo. Or calculate it here using the Harris-Benedict equation.

For women:

Take your weight in pounds and multiply it by 4.3: _____

Take your height in inches and multiply it by 4.7: _____

Add those two numbers together. _____

Then add 655: _____

This gives you subtotal A: _____

Now take your age and multiply it by 4.7: _____

This gives you subtotal B: _____

Now subtract subtotal B from subtotal A: _____

This is your BMR.

For men, the equation is different:

Take your weight in pounds and multiply it by 6.3: _____

Take your height in inches and multiply it by 12.9: _____

Add those two numbers together. _____

Then add 66: _____

This gives you subtotal A: _____

Now take your age and multiply it by 6.8: _____

This gives you subtotal B: _____

Now subtract subtotal B from subtotal A: _____

This is your BMR.

Example: a woman who is 140 pounds, 5 feet 5 inches, and 40 years old

Weight (140) × 4.3 = 602

Height in inches (65) × 4.7 = 305.5

Add those two numbers together, then add 655.

Subtotal A = 1,562.5

Age (40) × 4.7 = 188

Subtotal B = 188

Subtotal A (1,562.5) − Subtotal B (188) = 1,374.5 calories

Example: a man who is 180 pounds, 5 feet 10 inches, and 45 years old

Weight (180) × 6.3 = 1,134

Height in inches (70) × 12.9 = 903

Add those two numbers together, then add 66.

Subtotal A = 2,103

Age (45) × 6.8 = 306

Subtotal B = 306

Subtotal A (2,103) − Subtotal B (306) = 1,797 calories

Total Calories You Need to Maintain Your Current Weight

Now calculate the calories you use in a day, not including formal exercise.

If you are sedentary, multiply your BMR × 1.2.

If you are lightly active, multiply your BMR × 1.375.

If you are moderately active, multiply your BMR × 1.55.

If you are very active, multiply your BMR × 1.725.

If you are extra active, multiply your BMR × 1.9.

Enter the number here: _____

Continuing Weight Loss: Calories Out Must Exceed Calories In

In Week 4 of this workbook, you learned how many calories you're eating each day and how many calories you're burning each day through exercise. Adjusting those two variables gives you a blueprint for weight loss.

Let's see where you stand at the end of the running program. How many calories are you currently eating? Use the additional pages of food log starting on page 250 to log your food intake for at least 1 day and to calculate the calories in each of the foods you record. Sites like MyPyramid.gov, CalorieKing.com, and FitDay.com can help you determine the number of calories in the foods you're eating.

Current calorie intake: _____

Is this less than the number above, about the same, or more than the number above?

Exercise Plan

Many people find that after 12 weeks of careful eating, there aren't many places left to trim calories from their diet. So to continue losing weight, they have to exercise longer and harder.

Running, as we've shown, burns more calories than walking. Do the calculation below to see how many calories your average workout is burning now.

To get an accurate sense of your calorie burn for a typical workout, you need to know your distance. Try one workout on a measured course or around a track so you know how far you're going.

Take your body weight and multiply it by 0.53 to get the number of calories burned each time you walk 1 mile. Take your body weight and multiply it by 0.75 to get the number of calories you burn running 1 mile.

Weight _____ x 0.53 x _____ miles walked = _____ calories burned walking

Weight _____ x 0.75 x _____ miles run = _____ calories burned running

Add the two together: _____

Average workout burns _____ calories, multiplied by _____ workouts per week.

Weekly calorie deficit (calories saved from eating + calories burned while exercising): _____

Take that number and divide by 3,500: _____

This will result in continued weight loss of _____ pounds per week.

Goal Setting

Look again at the goals you set in Week 3 and revised in Week 7 of this workbook. If you've accomplished any of your goals, great! Now add a few new ones. Don't be complacent. Keep striving.

GOAL	DEADLINE FOR MEETING IT	HOW WILL YOU KNOW WHEN YOU'VE ACHIEVED YOUR GOAL?
1		
2		
3		
4		
5		
UPDATED GOALS		
1		
2		
3		
4		
5		

Food Log

TIME	WHERE ARE YOU EATING?	WHAT ARE YOU EATING?

Day   Date

HOW MUCH ARE YOU EATING?	ARE YOU HUNGRY (H) or NOT HUNGRY (NH)?	CALORIES	RATE YOUR DAY 1–5 1—Bad day 5—Great day

Food Log

TIME	WHERE ARE YOU EATING?	WHAT ARE YOU EATING?

Day _____   Date _____

HOW MUCH ARE YOU EATING?	ARE YOU HUNGRY (H) or NOT HUNGRY (NH)?	CALORIES	RATE YOUR DAY 1–5 1—Bad day 5—Great day

Food Log

TIME	WHERE ARE YOU EATING?	WHAT ARE YOU EATING?

Day   Date

HOW MUCH ARE YOU EATING?	ARE YOU HUNGRY (H) or NOT HUNGRY (NH)?	CALORIES	RATE YOUR DAY 1–5 1—Bad day 5—Great day

Food Log

TIME	WHERE ARE YOU EATING?	WHAT ARE YOU EATING?

Day _____   Date _____

HOW MUCH ARE YOU EATING?	ARE YOU HUNGRY (H) or NOT HUNGRY (NH)?	CALORIES	RATE YOUR DAY 1–5 1—Bad day 5—Great day

Food Log

TIME	WHERE ARE YOU EATING?	WHAT ARE YOU EATING?

Day   Date

HOW MUCH ARE YOU EATING?	ARE YOU HUNGRY (H) or NOT HUNGRY (NH)?	CALORIES	RATE YOUR DAY 1–5 1—Bad day 5—Great day

Food Log

TIME	WHERE ARE YOU EATING?	WHAT ARE YOU EATING?

Day   Date

HOW MUCH ARE YOU EATING?	ARE YOU HUNGRY (H) or NOT HUNGRY (NH)?	CALORIES	RATE YOUR DAY 1–5 1—Bad day 5—Great day

Food Log

TIME	WHERE ARE YOU EATING?	WHAT ARE YOU EATING?

Day   Date

HOW MUCH ARE YOU EATING?	ARE YOU HUNGRY (H) or NOT HUNGRY (NH)?	CALORIES	RATE YOUR DAY 1–5 1—Bad day 5—Great day

Food Log

TIME	WHERE ARE YOU EATING?	WHAT ARE YOU EATING?

Day   Date

HOW MUCH ARE YOU EATING?	ARE YOU HUNGRY (H) or NOT HUNGRY (NH)?	CALORIES	RATE YOUR DAY 1–5 1—Bad day 5—Great day

Exercise Log

DAY	TIME WALKING	TIME RUNNING	TOTAL WORKOUT TIME
MONDAY			
TUESDAY			
WEDNESDAY			
THURSDAY			
FRIDAY			
SATURDAY			
SUNDAY			

COURSE	NOTES (WEATHER, HOW YOU FELT, ETC.)	OTHER PHYSICAL ACTIVITY DURING THE DAY

Exercise Log

DAY	TIME WALKING	TIME RUNNING	TOTAL WORKOUT TIME
MONDAY			
TUESDAY			
WEDNESDAY			
THURSDAY			
FRIDAY			
SATURDAY			
SUNDAY			

COURSE	NOTES (WEATHER, HOW YOU FELT, ETC.)	OTHER PHYSICAL ACTIVITY DURING THE DAY

Exercise Log

DAY	TIME WALKING	TIME RUNNING	TOTAL WORKOUT TIME
MONDAY			
TUESDAY			
WEDNESDAY			
THURSDAY			
FRIDAY			
SATURDAY			
SUNDAY			

COURSE	NOTES (WEATHER, HOW YOU FELT, ETC.)	OTHER PHYSICAL ACTIVITY DURING THE DAY

Find out more on runnersworld.com

So you've caught the running bug and you want to learn more? Great! The editors of *Runner's World* love welcoming converts to the sport. The more, the merrier. And we've got information for you.

If you visit runnersworld.com, you'll find a wealth of articles for beginners planning their next moves. The site has training plans, nutrition advice, snack ideas, motivational videos, strength and flexibility routines, and suggestions for treating aches and pains, not to mention hilarious bloggers detailing the strange and wonderful things that happen in the lives of runners. If you need information on running, runnersworld.com is a one-stop shop.

A Weight-Loss Community

We're really excited about a new neighborhood within the site, runnersworld.com/rybo. It's a growing community of people who are starting to run with the goal of losing weight. The calculators in this book—for determining BMR, calories used in a day, and calories burned running and walking—are available there. We'll suggest great 5-Ks for beginners, and experts will be available to answer questions that pop up frequently from people who are new to running. Most important, we'll be spotlighting people who have successfully shed pounds through running.

Our test panelists and scores of other people who have lost weight tell us that accountability is a major component of their success. When you have the sense that someone is watching, and when you have to report your numbers to someone other than yourself, it's a lot easier to stick to your plans for fitness and eating. So check out the *RYBO* site, and share your experiences and progress with people who have the same goals you do. Or share your thoughts, feelings, and questions with us directly at Sarah@runyourbuttoffbook.com.

Acknowledgments

I am so grateful for my family, Fred, Greg, and Cary, for their support, brutal honesty, and love. A round of applause to our test panel and all my clients, who inspire and challenge me to guide them so they can attain and maintain their goals.

—*Leslie Bonci*

I'd like to thank my high school coach, Vince Mellon, for introducing me to running, and my mentor, Dee Coughlin, for teaching me to teach.

—*Budd Coates*

My gratitude first to Leslie Bonci and Budd Coates, whose expertise and experience made this book possible. They spent hours guiding our test panel by reading food logs, giving nutrition advice over the phone, and holding evening workouts and extra stretching sessions. They whipped me into shape, too. Leslie's advice helped me lose a few pounds, and Budd's workouts made me faster than I've been in a while. Thanks, Leslie and Budd. Let's do it again.

I got lucky with the people on the test panel—a fun, enthusiastic, and diligent group all around. I admire their courage in learning to run and in sharing their stories. They're no longer just participants in a study; they're friends. Thanks also to Michelle Sames for helping me find them.

My editors, John Atwood, Stephanie Knapp, and Shannon Welch, skillfully guided this book to the finish line. Joanna Sayago Golub, *Runner's World* senior editor, was a source of support and good cheer throughout, as was Amby Burfoot, *Runner's World* editor-at-large. Researchers

Sarah Eberspacher and Jordan Oliver were terrific at digging up obscure diet and exercise factoids at a moment's notice.

Thanks to my family and friends for their cheerleading during this project: Mom, Dan Lorge, Abigail Lorge, Claire Butler, Mark and Claire Bernstein, Amy and Judd Hark, Noreen Yamamoto and Vince Sherry, Carla Lindenmuth, Tricia Lipani, Darlene Sanderson, and Jess Walcott.

Finally, love to Charlie for your guidance, great ideas, and good humor, especially on Sunday afternoons. And to Leah and Ben, who demonstrate their version of *Run Your Butt Off!* with thunderous laps around the house: Thanks for making me laugh.

—*Sarah Lorge Butler*

Index

Boldface page references indicate photographs and illustrations. <u>Underscored</u> references indicate boxed text and charts.

C

CalorieKing.com, 73
Calories
  basal metabolic rate and, 14–16
  in breakfast, healthy, 50
  burning
    basal metabolic rate and, 14–16
    daily activities, 12
    running, 24, 28, 36, 104–5, 180–81
    walking, 28, 36
    workouts, 28
  counting
    attitude toward, 75–77
    Leslie's Lessons, 77
    for one day, 73–75, 74
    "one-quarter less rule" versus, 171
    resources, 73
    workbook and, personal, 74
  for current weight maintenance,
    determining, 16
  cutting, x, 75, 77
  daily need, xvi, 12, 12, 16, 17, 27
  deficit
    creating, xiv, 197
    for 1-pound weight loss per week,
     27, 29
    source of, **30**
    weight loss and, xvi, 105, 120, 197
  in fruits, 130
  Leslie's Lessons
    counting, 77
    cutting, 75
    daily need, 17
  protein and, 148–51, 149, 150
  in vegetables, 130
Carbohydrates, 145–46, 145
Cardiovascular conditioning, 11–12,
  102–3
Cereals, 72, 94, 163
Cheeses, 72, 164–66, 164
Chest measurement, 35
Chewing food, 108
Chicago Marathon (2010), ix–x
Children and eating habits, 194
Clothing, running, 8–9, 144
Condiments, 71–72
Consistency of workouts, xv, 41, 88, 143

Cooldown exercises, 44, **46–47**, 46–47
Core strength, building, **186–89**, 186–89
Cravings, food, 192, 193–95
Cross-training exercise, 43

D

Dairy products, 94. *See also specific type*
Daydreaming and running, 142–43, 142
Diet. *See also* Food; Food Talk
  boredom factor and, 166–69, 167, 169,
    194
  brain and, training for healthy, 72–73,
    90
  carbohydrates in, 144, 145–46
  children and, 194
  dietary fats in, 163–64
  dining out, 195–96
  eliminating category of food and,
    avoiding, 50–51
  exercise and, 29
  family barbecues and, 194–95
  fiber in, 128–29, 145, 162–63
  food colors and, 126–29, 127
  food shopping and, 90–94, 93, 127
  grazing and, avoiding, 55–56, 55, 170–71
  Happy Hours and, managing, 193–94
  kitchen pantry and, cleaning out,
    94–95
  meal planning and, 91–92
  meal scheduling and, 48, 48, 49
  meats in, 94, 165–66, 165
  overeating, 111
  packaged food in, 166
  protein in
    breakfast, 147
    calories and, 148–51, 149, 150
    dinner, 148
    drinks, 152
    Food Talk, 145
    increasing intake of, 145, 146–51, 150
    Leslie's Lessons, 146
    lunch, 147
    nutritional benefits of, 145–46, 145
    requirements, daily, 144–45
    snacks, 147–48
    type of, right, 146, 148–49

self-evaluation, 196, 197
sports drinks and, avoiding, 105–6
typical, for Leslie, 34
"uploading" and, 48
weekends versus weekdays and, 151, 153, 154
Dietary fats, 163–64
Dieting, xii–xiii, 72, 144, 163
Dining out, 195–96
Dinner
  family, 108
  fruits for, 129
  protein in, 148
  spicing up, 168
  vegetables for, 129
Distance, running, 158
Dynamic flexibility exercises, 44–47, 44–47

E

Eating habits
  changing, 33
  chewing food, 108
  children and, 194
  family barbecue, 195
  food log and, 30, 48
  Food Talk, 30, 48
  Happy Hours and, 193–94
  hunger and, 48, 56
  lifetime changes in, 169
  nighttime, 54–55, 54
  office snacks, 194
  portion control and, 71–73
  problems and solutions, common, 193–95
  slow eating, 106–10, 106
  of Test Panel, 196–97
  weight loss and, 30
Eating out, 195–96
Eating plan of RYBO program, xv
Endorphins, 101, 101
Energy expenditure, calculating, 27–29
Exercise. See also Running; Walking; Workouts
  benefits of, 89
  cooldown, 44, 46–47, 46–47
  core-strengthening, 186–89, 186–89
  cross-training, 43
  diet and, 29
  dynamic flexibility, 44–47, 44–47
  endorphins and, 101, 101
  hooked on, 100–101
  hunger after, 130–33
  log
    Amy W.'s, 6–7
    charts, 266–71
    Noel Carol's, 118–19
  stretching, 44–47, 44–47
  warmup, 44–46, 44–46
  weight loss and, 119–20
Exertion as ecstasy, 101
Experts, RYBO program, xvii, xvii. See also Budd's Buzz; Leslie's Lessons

F

Fad diets, 72, 144, 163
Family barbecues, 195
Family dinners, 108
Fat. See Body, fat; Dietary fats
Fiber, 127, 145, 162–63
First Strides (running program), 64, 100, 138
5-K races, 82–83, 178, 181–82
Food. See also Diet; specific type
  changes, personal, 190
  chewing, 108
  choices, 173
  colors, 126–29, 127
  cravings, 192, 193–95
  flavor in, 163–64
  fresh versus canned, 129
  labels, 70, 72–73
  log
    charts, 250–65
    creating, 30–31, 185
    Dorene's, 190, 190–91, 192
    after Easter, 95
    eating habits and, 30, 48
    Food Talk, 30
    importance of, 30–31
    Leslie's, 34, 76, 76
    privacy and, 32–33

breakfast, 50
calories
   counting, 77
   cutting, 75
   daily need, 17
cheeses, 164
cravings, food, 192
eating habits, 33
exercise and diet, 29
family dinners, 108
food choices, 173
food log, 95
food measurements, 71
food shopping, 93
fresh versus canned fruits and
   vegetables, 129
goal-setting, 57
grazing, 55
hunger, 171
meats, 165
nighttime eating habits, 54
overeating, 111
protein, 146
rewards after running, 111
run/reward cycle, 111, 113
self-talk, 198
weekend versus weekday diet and,
   154
weight gain, 110
Logs
   exercise
      Amy W.'s, 6–7
      charts, 266–71
      Noel Carol's, 118–19
   food
      charts, 250–65
      creating, 30–31, 185
      Dorene's, 190, 190–91, 192
      after Easter, 95
      eating habits and, 30, 48
      Food Talk, 30
      importance of, 30–31
      Leslie's, 34, 76, 76
      privacy and, 32–33
      purposes, 31–32

      Sarah's, 149–51, 149, 150
      using, 216, 216–17
Long runs, 182–84, 185
Lunch
   fruits for, 128–29
   protein in, 147
   spicing up, 168
   vegetables for, 128–29

M

Meals. *See also specific meal*
   planning, 91–92
   scheduling, 48, 48, 49
Measurements
   body, 35
   body weight, 27
   chest, 35
   food, 70, 71–72
   hip, 35
   thigh, 35
   waist, 35
Meats, 94, 165–66, 165
Milk, 94, 106
"Moisture-wicking" fabrics, 8
Motivation
   Budd's Buzz, 144
   compliments on weight loss, 160–61
   racing, 82
   running, 102–3, 158–59, 160–61
Muscle-building, 12, 23
Music and running, 159
MyPyramid.gov, 73

N

Negative self-talk, avoiding, 198
Nighttime eating, 54–55, 54

O

Oatmeal, 166
Office snacks, 194
"One-quarter less" rule and calories, 171
Overeating, 111